# PRAISE FOR DR. LINDSEY

*Dr. Lindsey's expertise in the orthodontic field moved my teeth, improved my smile, and more importantly increased my confidence. His passion for helping others achieve this increased self-esteem through a great smile spilled over to influence and change my life forever. Now, I have the honor of treating my own patients with the respect and care that Dr. Lindsey did for me, and I can't imagine a better field in which to work and serve!*

**—Emily F. Howell, DMD**

*This is a most charming writing. Dustin Burleson does book writing and follows Dan Kennedy's marketing principles. But you are far better than he. My compliments.*

**—Orhan Tuncay, DMD**, Rittenhouse Orthodontics, author of *The Invisalign System*

*Having consulted with over seven hundred orthodontic practices, I have a nationwide perspective of a "peak performance practice." Dr. Lindsey is an extremely progressive clinician. He is an excellent boss and retains very talented team members. I admire Dr. Lindsey's compassion and dedication to his family, patients, team, and referring doctors. I have been fortunate to have Dr. Lindsey as a client for many years.*

**—Charlene White,** world-renowned orthodontic consultant, owner of Progressive Concepts, Inc.

# IMAGINE

## YOUR BEST SMILE

DR. CHARLES LINDSEY

# IMAGINE
## YOUR BEST SMILE

### HOW ORTHODONTICS CAN CHANGE
### –AND EVEN SAVE–YOUR LIFE

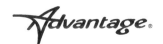

Published by Advantage, Charleston, South Carolina.
Member of Advantage Media Group.

ADVANTAGE is a registered trademark, and the Advantage colophon is a trademark of Advantage Media Group, Inc.

Printed in the United States of America.

10  9  8  7  6  5  4  3  2  1

ISBN: 978-1-642250-52-7
LCCN: 2019912328

Book design by Megan Elger.

This publication is designed to provide accurate and authoritative information in regard to the subject matter covered. It is sold with the understanding that the publisher is not engaged in rendering legal, accounting, or other professional services. If legal advice or other expert assistance is required, the services of a competent professional person should be sought.

Advantage Media Group is proud to be a part of the Tree Neutral® program. Tree Neutral offsets the number of trees consumed in the production and printing of this book by taking proactive steps such as planting trees in direct proportion to the number of trees used to print books. To learn more about Tree Neutral, please visit **www.treeneutral.com**.

Advantage Media Group is a publisher of business, self-improvement, and professional development books and online learning. We help entrepreneurs, business leaders, and professionals share their Stories, Passion, and Knowledge to help others Learn & Grow. Do you have a manuscript or book idea that you would like us to consider for publishing? Please visit **advantagefamily.com** or call **1.866.775.1696**.

*To my beautiful wife, Shea, for her endless support and patience during my many hours devoted to writing this book.*

# CONTENTS

ABOUT THE AUTHOR . . . . . . . . . . . . . . . xi

ACKNOWLEDGMENTS . . . . . . . . . . . . . xiii

INTRODUCTION . . . . . . . . . . . . . . . . . 1
**ORTHODONTICS GAVE ME A LIFE-CHANGING SMILE**

CHAPTER ONE . . . . . . . . . . . . . . . . . 9
**ORTHODONTICS FOR A BETTER SMILE—A BETTER YOU**

CHAPTER TWO . . . . . . . . . . . . . . . . . 21
**THE ART AND SCIENCE OF MOVING TEETH**

CHAPTER THREE . . . . . . . . . . . . . . . . 33
**THE "TOOLS" I USE FOR MOVING TEETH**

CHAPTER FOUR . . . . . . . . . . . . . . . . 55
**INVISALIGN CLEAR ALIGNER THERAPY— A NEW WORLD OF ORTHODONTICS**

CHAPTER FIVE . . . . . . . . . . . . . . . . . 65
**DIFFERENT TREATMENTS AT EVERY AGE— EARLY AND ADOLESCENT TREATMENT**

CHAPTER SIX . . . . . . . . . . . . . . . . . 77
**TREATMENT FOR ADULTS**

CHAPTER SEVEN . . . . . . . . . . . . . . . . . . . 85
## RETAINING YOUR SMILE

CHAPTER EIGHT . . . . . . . . . . . . . . . . . . . 93
## A BETTER EXPERIENCE

CHAPTER NINE . . . . . . . . . . . . . . . . . . . 101
## GIVING BACK

CONCLUSION . . . . . . . . . . . . . . . . . . . 109

APPENDIX . . . . . . . . . . . . . . . . . . . 111

GLOSSARY . . . . . . . . . . . . . . . . . . . 113

OUR SERVICES . . . . . . . . . . . . . . . . . . . 119

# ABOUT THE AUTHOR

When it comes to orthodontics, Charles Lindsey, DMD, is a lifelong learner. A native of Georgia, Dr. Lindsey graduated from the Medical College of Georgia and completed his orthodontic residency at the University of Kentucky in Lexington. Since then, he has continually educated himself and his team on the latest advances in orthodontic treatment. Having undergone a number of dental and orthodontic procedures himself, Dr. Lindsey also has a rare insight into his patients' needs and wants.

Today, his orthodontic practice encompasses offices in Griffin and Locust Grove, Georgia. In these areas, Dr. Lindsey is the top provider of Invisalign clear aligner therapy for straightening teeth. Together, Dr. Lindsey and his team are devoted to making a positive difference in patients' lives by helping them overcome hurdles to achieving a life-changing smile.

Dr. Lindsey gives back to his communities through youth scholarships and free dental care for select individuals. He also uses his skills as a pilot to encourage youth to pursue careers in aviation, to provide free rides during an annual patient appreciation day, and to transport patients in need of medical care through the Angel Flight organization.

# ACKNOWLEDGMENTS

I have been blessed with many wonderful people throughout my life who helped me to make a career in orthodontics. Certainly, I couldn't have picked more supportive and helpful parents, who always encouraged me to be my best. I had the opportunity to learn from some of the best educators in the fields of engineering, dentistry, and orthodontics. However, I've learned far more while working with the many wonderful patients that I've had the great honor of treating these many years. Most of all, I am grateful to my spiritual Father who made everything possible.

# ORTHODONTICS GAVE ME A LIFE-CHANGING SMILE

When I tell my patients what it's like to undergo orthodontic treatment, it's more than doctorly experience I'm sharing. I really know what it's like to be in their shoes. You see, as someone who has had a number of dental and orthodontic challenges, I've undergone—and continue to undergo—many of the treatments that I now perform on patients.

At an early age, I learned that I was missing several permanent teeth in the front of my smile: two on top and two on the bottom. While it wasn't easy living with so many missing teeth, it didn't really begin to bother me until I was a preteen. At that point, I began to be very self-conscious of how my mouth looked. I wouldn't smile for pictures or, if I did smile, I'd keep my lips together. I didn't want people to see that I had so many missing teeth; I didn't want a permanent record of those gaps. Over time, my teeth began to affect my personality. I became very shy and introverted because I was so self-conscious about how my teeth looked.

I grew up in a middle-class family near Atlanta, Georgia. My dad was a maintenance foreman for Eastern Airlines and my mother was a registered nurse. I was extremely fortunate to have parents that made it a priority to provide dental and orthodontic care to correct my oral problems. Back then, implants were in the early stages of development and basically not available to replace my missing teeth. Instead, I wore braces to put all my teeth into the proper positions and to open up even more space for replacement teeth. Then my dentist created bridges, which comprised replacement "teeth" that are held in place in my mouth with crowns on either side of the gaps. Today, I still have two bridges on top and one on the bottom.

I also had an overjet, which is a condition where my lower jaw didn't grow as much as the upper jaw. Today, we can quite often correct the condition with amazing results using orthodontic appliances, which can help a patient's lower jaw to grow forward. But back then, there really wasn't any treatment or technology to fully correct the problem. So, my orthodontist did the best he could but, until I was an adult, I had an overjet and a deficient lower jaw. Then, after I graduated from orthodontic residency at age thirty, I put braces back on and had orthognathic surgery to move my lower jaw forward. Just before I began writing this book, I also started Invisalign clear aligner therapy to get a broader smile that wasn't addressed with orthodontic treatment when I was young. With Invisalign, I also wanted to better understand the treatments I'm offering my patients, so now I know what that experience is like as well.

While the surgery improved my facial structure, and Invisalign is improving my smile, it was orthodontic treatment as a youth that made the greatest impact on my life. Once it was complete, my life changed dramatically. I went from barely smiling, or hiding my teeth with closed lips, to smiling a big, broad smile all the time. But this didn't happen overnight. My picture on the right was taken shortly after completing orthodontic treatment, but I wasn't quite ready to smile big for the camera. Soon my new smile really did help me open up as a person—I was no longer concerned about people seeing my teeth, so I became much more outgoing and confident. Within a year, I had my first girlfriend and became the starting pitcher on the high school baseball team.

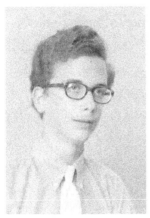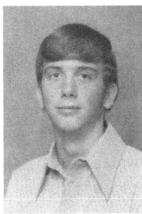

*This is me at thirteen and fifteen years old, before and after orthodontic treatment. My new smile not only changed my teeth but inspired me to get contacts and do something with that hair.*

In fact, my life was so changed by treatment that I decided to make a career of helping other people that had less-than-ideal smiles. At age fifteen, I became so interested in orthodontics that I began pursuing it as a career. You see, I loved my dentist. He did a lot of great work in restoring my missing teeth. But I noticed a major difference in the atmosphere between the dentist's and orthodontist's offices. Specifically, the orthodontist's office was more worry-free, a bit friendlier, and on some levels, actually fun. I thought it seemed like a great career to help people improve their lives through their smile and have fun while doing it.

Today, thirty years and thousands of patients later, I've seen orthodontics make the same kind of difference in the lives of many people as it made in mine.

## An Atypical Career Path—for an Orthodontist

My career path was a little atypical. After graduating from high school, I knew I wanted to become an orthodontist, but I didn't know if I would actually be accepted into dental school, since there's a pretty stringent admission process. As a backup plan of sorts, in college, I majored in something else that I was also interested in— engineering. I knew that if my dream of being an orthodontist didn't work out, I could have a fulfilling career as an engineer. My dad often dealt with engineers in his role as a troubleshooter with the airline, and he had a lot of respect for them. Since I excelled in math in high school, my dad helped steer me toward engineering when he saw that I was somewhat undecided about a major in college.

Ultimately, I really enjoyed studying engineering, but after three years in college, I still wanted a career as an orthodontist. My friends thought I was crazy for wanting to continue on with school for as long as it would take, but I was determined. I applied to dental school, which required me to take more courses in biology and chemistry— all this helped me get accepted into dental school. After I graduated, with a bachelor's in mechanical engineering from Georgia Tech, I went to the Medical College of Georgia to receive a doctorate of dental medicine. Then, I completed an orthodontic residency at the University of Kentucky. Still, I was glad I had pursued a mechanical engineering degree, because it actually provided a very good background for orthodontics. It helped me better understand the complicated vectors, forces, and materials involved in moving and aligning teeth.

Eleven years after graduating high school, I went to work as an orthodontist. My first job was in an existing practice in Gainesville, Georgia, where I worked for about eighteen months. The orthodontist that owned the practice wanted to reduce his workload, so he sold me his satellite office in northeast Georgia. Ten years later, I moved to Atlanta and started the practice I'm in today. Along the way, I've also worked as an associate for other orthodontists as a great way of gaining insights into treating patients.

It's been an interesting road, being both an orthodontist and a businessman. And it all started with getting treatment for my own smile.

## A Lot Has Changed

About twenty years ago, I was having lunch with a referring dentist and he asked me, "So what's new in orthodontics?" I thought about it for a few minutes and really had no answer for him. Not much had really changed back then. Today, I'd be able to talk for hours about all that's going on in orthodontics—that's how much has changed. Orthodontics today is a rapidly changing treatment, making the movement of teeth more comfortable and esthetic and, in some cases, faster.

*Orthodontics today is a rapidly changing treatment, making the movement of teeth more comfortable and esthetic and, in some cases, faster.*

One of the big developments in recent years is clear aligner therapy, what most people know as Invisalign. Clear aligners allow us to align people's teeth and create beautiful smiles without using metal braces. That means a lot more people are seeking orthodontic treatment, because they no longer have to wear a mouthful of metal to get a prettier smile or straighter teeth. Invisalign has become such an integral part of orthodontic treatment that I've devoted a whole chapter to the topic (chapter 4).

I used to offer lingual braces, which are bonded to the back of the teeth and virtually invisible from the front. But one of the main complaints was that they interfered with the patient's speech. Invisalign has become a very good alternative to lingual braces because the aligners are not very noticeable and they don't cause changes in your speech as is common with lingual braces.

There are a lot of other advances in orthodontics that have improved everything from diagnosis to treatment to retention.

For instance, cone beam technology now allows us to take 3-D x-ray images of patients that give us a view into their structures of the mouth and face. The cone beam allows me to identify issues ranging from impacted teeth to obstructed airways, while helping expand the types of treatment I'm able to offer patients.

Impressions are also a thing of the past in my practice. Today, we have a scanner that takes a video image of the teeth, which is digitally manipulated on a computer screen to help with treatment planning. We can also use this to help patients visualize their new smile. When used with a 3-D printer, the scanning technology allows us to create retainers in-house same-day or overnight. We don't always need to have the retainers made this quickly, but it is nice to have that option when it is necessary.

I also have a diode laser, a tool that lets me perform some procedures in-office without the patient having to be treated by an oral surgeon.

These technologies, and others, help make patients' lives easier and less complex. I'll talk about these developments more in-depth in chapter 2.

## Flying High

Today, my life is soaring—literally. While I love being able to help patients through my skills and experience as an orthodontist, flying was really my first passion. In fact, at a very early age, I wanted a career in aviation. But at age seven, I found out that I was nearsighted, which ruled out a career as an airline pilot. Still, after my first ride in a private airplane at age twenty, I was hooked—I thought it was like being in a convertible going 115 miles per hour.

After that, I took flying lessons through Georgia Tech's Flying Club and received my pilot's license. I've been airborne as often as possible ever since.

In addition to flying my family on our vacations, I've flown all over the United States and to the Caribbean, logging roughly 2,600 hours to date and earning single-engine, multi-engine, seaplane, commercial, instrument, and instructor ratings. I don't currently teach, but earning an instructor rating required me to learn so much more about flying, and it has made me a safer, more confident pilot.

I love flying so much that I use my ability for the good of others. I'm a pilot for Angel Flight, an organization that flies patients in need to medical treatment a long distance away. I'm involved with Young Eagles, a chapter of the Experimental Aircraft Association that encourages an interest in aviation in youth. And every year, my practice has a Patient Appreciation Day where I take people on a plane ride, often their first. I'll talk more about my high-flying adventures—and other ways the practice gives back—in chapter 9.

That's really what it's all about—giving back to patients. I want to always give them more in use value than they give me in cash value. Using my knowledge and expertise, I want to add more value to their personal and professional lives—many, many times more value—than the fees that I charge.

Through my own experiences with orthodontic treatment, and in my everyday encounters with patients, I really feel I'm doing that. After all, that's why I became an orthodontist—I wanted others to feel the same elation that I felt all those years ago, and that I still feel at the end of every treatment. I want patients to look in the mirror at the end of treatment and see what a life-changing difference ortho-dontics makes.

# CHAPTER ONE

# ORTHODONTICS FOR A BETTER SMILE—A BETTER YOU

Imagine what it's like to wake up every day and greet the world with your best smile. Maybe you have an upcoming event, a big presentation at work, a first date—even a neighborhood barbecue. Imagine how much happier, how much more confident you would be if you were wearing the smile you had always dreamed of having.

With today's advances in orthodontic treatment, you can have that smile and be a healthier, more confident you.

I feel confident making that claim because, in the more than three decades that I've been treating patients, I've seen how orthodontics can be a life-changing experience. Patients that come to see me for treatment often start out as shy introverts—with less-than-ideal smiles. Sometimes they don't smile at all, and it can be a challenge to get them to even open up and tell me about the problems in their mouth—even though I specialize in creating beautiful smiles.

But when we get to work on their smile, they begin to open up and really become the person they always were inside. They open up to me, and they open up to the world, once they have a smile they're proud to show.

*When we get to work on their smile, they begin to open up and really become the person they always were inside.*

The transformation for many patients is really nothing short of amazing. Peyton is a great example of what I'm talking about. When she first came in, her hair was disheveled, and she was crying. Her past experiences with dental treatment had been unhappy ones, so she was very afraid of having any type of orthodontic treatment. She was also very shy—we could hardly get her to talk.

Even though she had not gone through treatment a few years earlier, which would have taken advantage of her growing jaws and corrected many of the problems she was now facing, we felt that we could still help her have the smile her parents had imagined for her.

Since she was an adolescent, most of Peyton's permanent teeth were in when I first saw her. Those that weren't would likely have impacted, or remained under the tissue in her mouth, causing her unsightly teeth for the rest of her life without treatment. Fortunately, we found those kinds of problems and were able to put her in braces to make room for the rest of her permanent teeth, and then were able to guide those teeth into place. She also had a lot of crowding of the permanent teeth that were already in, so a number of them were crooked. I used her braces to align those crooked teeth and give Peyton her best smile.

Over the course of treatment, we'd spend our appointments with her talking about all the things that were important in her life: school, her birthday, her family, and the friendships she was beginning to form. As her teeth straightened, we noticed her confidence growing.

After Peyton's treatment was complete and the braces were removed, I brought her parents back to the treatment room and we all looked at her "before" pictures alongside her new smile. The results were amazing. Even I had not realized what a dramatic difference there was in her smile—in her total demeanor—until I saw her "before" pictures. She seemed to walk two feet taller, was outgoing with everyone, and smiled a big smile when we took her "after" photos.

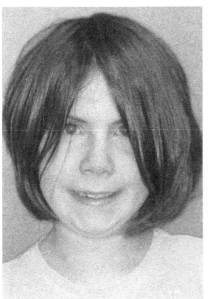 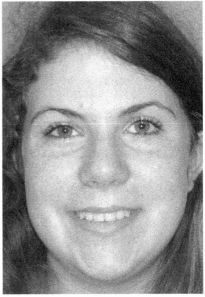

Peyton started treatment when she was eleven, but she looked like she was eight or nine at the time—that's how withdrawn and nervous she was. At the close of treatment two years later, she looked every bit the confident thirteen-year-old that she was. She had blossomed into a different person all together. "She's a different child now," her mom told us. "She's involved in all kinds of activities at school, where before, she didn't want anything to do with school at all."

As I shared in the introduction, my experience was very similar to Peyton's. You see, I'm an orthodontist, but I'm also a patient. Since adolescence, I've undergone several treatments to correct problems with my own smile and bite. From wearing braces and having bridges placed as a teen to correct genetically missing teeth, to undergoing jaw surgery as an adult to correct a bite discrepancy, to wearing Invisalign clear aligners to broaden my smile, I know what's it's like to imagine a better smile—and better functioning mouth—and then, through orthodontic treatment, see those dreams become reality.

That's my mission in life: to create the best smile for every patient that I see through orthodontics and to see their life change as a result of that treatment.

## Your Best Smile—Your Best Asset

A new smile is far more than just straight teeth. It really is your best asset. And obtaining your best smile can be a life-changing experience. As Peyton's story demonstrates (and mine, as I shared in the introduction), a better smile improves self-esteem and self-confidence. It can help you get into better schools, get a better job, make you more attractive to others, improve your health, and even save your life. There are a number of studies that prove my points.

A perception study for Invisalign, the maker of clear aligners that are often used to straighten teeth today (see chapter 4), asked participants to give their impressions after looking at photos of people—some with straight teeth, others with crooked teeth or other issues. According to the study:[1]

- Twenty-nine percent said that teeth were the first part of the face that they noticed.

- Twenty-four percent said teeth were the part of the face they remembered most.

- Forty-five percent thought that straight teeth would help a person land a job over another individual with crooked teeth.

- Seventy-three percent thought that those people with nice smiles were more trustworthy.

More than half (57 percent) of the people in another study cited overall hygiene as their top must-have when it comes to looking for a partner.[2]

As a confidence-builder, a Harris Poll found that, of two thousand people surveyed:[3]

- Sixty-three percent believe confidence equates to happiness.

- Seventy-eight percent said that having their teeth straightened gave them the confidence to tackle something they had not tried before.

---

1   "First Impressions Are Everything: New Study Confirms People With Straight Teeth Are Perceived as More Successful, Smarter and Having More Dates," PR Newswire, Apr 19, 2012, accessed April 26, 2018, 2018, https://www.prnewswire.com/news-releases/first-impressions-are-everything-new-study-confirms-people-with-straight-teeth-are-perceived-as-more-successful-smarter-and-having-more-dates-148073735.html.

2   Sharon Jayson, "What singles want: Survey looks at attraction, turnoffs," USA Today, February 5, 2013, accessed June 20, 2018, https://www.usatoday.com/story/news/nation/2013/02/04/singles-dating-attraction-facebook/1878265.

3   "New survey reveals how teeth straightening impacts overall confidence," Invisalign, news release, May 18, 2016, accessed August 31, 2018, https://www.invisalign.com/news-and-events/2016/invisalign-national-survey-results-released.

- Fifty-seven percent rate teeth as the second reason for their insecurity, behind weight.

Studies show that people that smile a lot live longer. One study that simply looked at the longevity of baseball players from an old photo found a seven-year difference in lifespan between those that smiled big and those that didn't smile at all.[4] Smiling can certainly lower stress levels, and that's definitely a way to improve one's health. As I shared in the introduction, I'm proof of more self-confidence and a much happier life since I had my smile fixed as a child.

Certainly, like my mom and dad, parents want their kids to have happy, stress-free childhoods. Yet, it's an unfortunate fact of life that unattractive teeth may even make a child the target of bullies.[5] People with poorly aligned teeth, gaps, crooked teeth, or other problems in the mouth are often viewed in a lesser light. Sometimes, I perform early treatment to try ward off bullying of a child that is self-conscious about being teased and mistreated because of the condition of their teeth. Some of the treatments I offer can improve their appearance, while also addressing the functional issues of their mouth. That can help them socially on a couple of levels: one, it can begin to correct problems early, rather than waiting for adolescence, when all their permanent teeth have come in, and two, it shows others that they care enough about their teeth to do something about the problems.

I'll talk more about early treatment for children and treatment for adolescents in chapter 5.

---

4    "Why You'll Live Longer By Smiling," Colgate, accessed August 30, 2018, https://www.colgate.com/en-in/oral-health/cosmetic-dentistry/teeth-whitening/why-you-ll-live-longer-by-smiling-more.

5    Débora Lopes Salles Scheffel et al., "Esthetic dental anomalies as motive for bullying in schoolchildren," *European Journal of Dentistry* 8, no. 1 (January–March 2014): 124-128, https://doi.org/10.4103/1305-7456.126266.

Adults often seek treatment after having to forgo it as a child. Since their parents couldn't afford to provide them with orthodontic treatment, they often look to correct issues they've had their whole lives, now that they have more disposable income. For some, it's a matter of putting their child's teeth first. I practice in a very blue-collar area, so for some, it's a matter of ensuring their children get the treatment they need first, and then coming in for treatment for themselves. I'll talk more about the complexities of treating adult teeth in chapter 6.

The truth is, we're living in a time when appearance is becoming a priority. We're beyond selfie-awareness as a fad, and since social media almost guarantees you will be seen, people are looking for ways to improve their looks. In fact, plastic surgeons have reported an uptick in patients looking for temporary procedures like Botox, reportedly because they want to look better in selfies.[6] Whether you want to or not—and smiling or not—there's a good chance you're going to appear online.

## A Smile Can Save Your Life

In addition to looking better, people with straight teeth also tend to have healthier mouths and better health overall.

Malocclusion, also known as a bad bite, is when the teeth do not properly meet during a bite because there are too many crooked, crowded, or misaligned teeth, or because the jaws did not grow in unison.

---

6    "Social Media Makes Lasting Impact on Industry – Becomes Cultural Force, Not Fad," American Academy of Facial Plastic and Reconstructive Surgery, Inc., news release, January 29, 2018, https://www.aafprs.org/media/stats_polls/m_stats. html.

A bad bite can cause uneven wear on teeth and even lead to chipping or fractures in teeth. That can lead to a host of problems requiring time in the dentist's chair.

Straight, aligned teeth without gaps are also easier to clean, meaning fewer incidences of tooth decay and gum disease. In fact, teeth and gums need to be in good condition to undergo orthodontic treatment. Often, people that come in for orthodontic treatment haven't been to a dentist in some time. Before we begin orthodontics, we sometimes have to get the patient back on track with regular visits to their dentist, or may even refer them to a periodontist to address gum issues or periodontal disease.

A bad bite can even create problems with the jaw joints, a condition known as temporomandibular joint dysfunction (TMJ or TMD). Patients with TMJ often experience symptoms such as morning headaches and chronic jaw pain, because their malocclusion can cause them to clench and grind their teeth, known as bruxism. Orthodontics can correct a bad bite and alleviate problems with malocclusion. Orthodontists can also provide what's known as a night guard, or splint, to cushion the teeth from the damaging effects of clenching and grinding.

When an adult patient with TMJ comes to see me, I sometimes steer them toward Invisalign clear aligner treatment. In addition to straightening their teeth, Invisalign clear aligners provide two layers of plastic that help cushion the teeth from the damaging effects of clenching and grinding.

One patient of mine, Stella, was in her sixties when she came in to have her teeth straightened. She also had been having TMJ pain for a number of years, so I treated her with Invisalign. Then, I put her in retainers that are similar to Invisalign once her teeth were straightened. Her TMJ symptoms immediately subsided as soon as she began treatment and they have never returned. Invisalign and retainer therapy gave Stella the smile she had always imagined, and as an added bonus worked well for her TMJ. At times, I see patients that have particularly bad TMJ, and I refer them to a local dentist that has great success in treating such cases.

In addition to better oral function and hygiene, straight teeth can actually help you be healthier overall.

There are orthodontic treatments today that can actually help prevent or alleviate obstructive sleep apnea (OSA), a disorder in which breathing stops periodically during sleep. This can cause a multitude of physical problems, from just being sleepy during the day to actually falling asleep while driving, along with other serious problems such as hypertension, obesity, diabetes, and cardiac disease. OSA is caused by an obstruction in the airway, anywhere from the tip of the nose to the back of the throat. That obstruction can be caused by issues such as enlarged tonsils or adenoids, for which I refer patients to an ear, nose, and throat specialist (ENT). Or, the obstruction may be the result of the patient not having enough room in their mouth for their tongue to rest comfortably. When there's not enough room for the tongue, it can relax back into the throat during sleep, causing an obstruction of the airway. Through orthodontics, I can move teeth and provide more room for the tongue, so it doesn't end up in blocking the airway and producing OSA.

Today, we have the technology to better detect the source of such problems. I'll discuss these technologies, OSA, and advances in orthodontics in the chapters ahead.

Besides OSA, poor oral health is connected to poor overall health.

Research has found links between oral hygiene and heart disease stemming from gum conditions such as gingivitis or periodontal disease. When the gums are unhealthy, the bacteria that live there can enter the bloodstream and cause damaging inflammation, which can raise the risk of problems with the heart and arteries, potentially leading to a heart attack or stroke.[7]

I've shared with you a lot of studies to support how a better smile leads to a better overall you. But I don't need any studies to know what I've seen for myself: Once treatment is complete, most patients tend to take pride in their new smile. They brush and floss regularly, and, in general, have better oral health. That can mean better health overall—and a better overall you.

## Now's the Time

The cost of orthodontics is as affordable as ever. Compared to others of life's needs and wants, the cost of orthodontic treatment has not comparatively increased over time.

Today, as I write these words, an average treatment plan still costs about what it did ten years ago. It used to be a yearly thing to up the cost of treatment a few percentage points—just like every other cost in life. But in my own practice, I have not had to do that.

*Improved technologies have vastly improved efficiencies with treatment, which helps to keep costs down.*

Improved technologies have vastly improved efficiencies with treatment, which helps to keep costs down. Because of those efficiencies, patients don't have to come as often for their adjustments, yet their treatment is still completed in the same amount of

---

7    Tracey Sandilands, "How Oral Health and Heart Disease Are Connected," Colgate, accessed March 3, 2018, https://www.colgate.com/en-us/oral-health/conditions/heart-disease/how-oral-health-and-heart-disease-are-connected-0115.

time as in the past. With Invisalign, for instance, I have lower lab fees because of the number of patients I'm able to treat. Those lower costs are passed on to patients. Plus, I have a great staff that assists with administration, finances, and some areas of clinical care, leaving me to concentrate on each patient's treatment plan and progress.

To make treatment affordable for anyone, there are a number of payment plans available (I'll discuss these more in-depth in chapter 8). What's important to remember is this: Orthodontics is one of the best investments to be made at any age. Yes, it's an investment in better-looking teeth, and in better health. But it's also an investment in peace of mind, and a better future. We often have patients come in for a second opinion after having been to another office with lower fees. Although the fee there may be lower, often what's lacking is the kind of personalized care, and even the quality of treatment, that we deliver at my office. And it's a little painful for everyone involved when a patient has to undergo retreatment because they are unhappy with the results of their first treatment.

The chapters ahead were written to inform you about your options and to let you know that there are orthodontic solutions today that can create a beautiful—and healthy—smile. *Your best smile.*

# CHAPTER TWO

# THE ART AND SCIENCE OF MOVING TEETH

In baseball, players often choose a bat they feel is special when it's their turn up to the plate. With one swing of the bat, they hit the ball out of the park. But as anyone watching the game knows, it's not the Louisville slugger that hits the home run, it's the player behind the bat.

*It's not the tools that do a great job of straightening teeth, it's the expertise of the orthodontist behind the tools that makes all the difference.*

The same concept holds true for orthodontics. When it comes to straightening teeth, it's often believed that a certain kind of braces or Invisalign clear aligners is what creates a beautiful smile. But those are only tools. And it's not the tools that do a great job of straightening teeth, it's the expertise of the orthodontist behind the tools that makes all the difference. It takes a skilled orthodontist, equipped with knowledge about the art and science of moving teeth, to get great results. The best smiles come from having an experienced orthodontist with the training and tools to determine the specifics of smile components, but who also knows how to look at a patient and visually gauge their individual needs.

Emily Howell is someone who saw how the skill and experience behind the tools can change a person's life. When Emily was a freshman in high school, she had a gap between her two front teeth that made her embarrassed to smile—so she rarely did. Then, her parents brought her in for treatment and I put her in braces that closed the gap, straightened the rest of her teeth, and gave her what would turn out to be a winning smile.

A few years after treatment, Emily became Miss Georgia 2001, and one year later, she competed in the Miss America 2002 pageant.

Perhaps even more exciting was Emily's future after she was crowned. She was so impacted by her own treatment that she decided to become an orthodontist herself. She wanted to make a difference in other peoples' lives by helping them change their smile and have newfound confidence. Today, Emily Howell, DMD, has a thriving practice, which has been recognized as one of the fastest-growing in the United States and a "reader's choice" in the county where she practices.

## The Artistry of the Smile

To determine what's best for each patient and give their smile an artistic edge, I analyze three factors: their whole face, their smile, and their teeth and gums.

**The whole face**. As orthodontists, we're not just treating the teeth; we're also treating the face. That's a different mindset than in the past—orthodontists used to believe that the teeth were the most important feature to address in creating a better smile. But then it was found that, even when the teeth were straightened, the face was still not as attractive as it could be in some people.

Today, we look at the whole face when we diagnose a patient and initiate their treatment plan. When looking at the whole face, I look at the relationship between the nose, lips, and chin. I look at the fullness of the face, because what is done with the teeth can either improve the profile relationship, or it can take away from it. The profile is basically a view of the face from the side, and the relationship involves looking at that shape from the forehead to the chin.

Over time, the facial profile changes as a result of the natural aging process—the nose and chin continue to grow larger, but the lips do not. When the lips aren't positioned forward enough, compared to the nose and chin, the face appears older. In the past, extractions used to be more common to make room for all the teeth in the mouth. But that took away from the profile by moving everything back, including the underlying bone structure for the lips. Orthodontic treatment today looks at bringing or keeping the structures of the mouth forward to give the tissues of the face the support they need to look more youthful, even as the rest of the body ages.

There's a concept known as the "Golden Proportion," which uses mathematical calculations to determine ideal dimensions between all the components of the face as a way of defining beauty. While the Golden Proportion serves as a good guideline, each patient is an individual and facial structures vary from patient to patient. Age, race, ethnicity, gender—all of these and more make for different profiles, so what works for one person may not be ideal for another. Some people have large teeth, some have small teeth, some have different jaw relationships. Missing teeth. Extra teeth. All of these factors must be taken into account when determining what can be done for a patient. While I start with certain guidelines and aim for certain goals, I must also determine how close we can get to ideal with each individual patient. Perfection is not always achievable, but what we can end up with is something that is far from where we started—and a very life-changing outcome.

That's the point of imagining *your* best smile, because the best smile for you is not the best smile for someone else. It's the best smile for you—it's the best smile for your face. That's where the artistry comes in.

**The smile**. In the smile, I look at factors such as the smile arc, or the curve of the smile (think happy face versus sad face). In the past, orthodontic treatment focused on making the bottom edges of the upper teeth appear as a straight line across. But that made the smile look somewhat manufactured.

A more pleasing appearance is when the smile creates an arc where the upper incisors (the four teeth in the center) follow the curvature of the lower lip. It takes training, experience—and a bit of artistry—to know how to position the brackets on the teeth or create an Invisalign treatment plan to produce that more natural-looking end result.

**The teeth and gums**. Clearly, the alignment of the teeth is important. But so is the shape and size of each tooth, and their size and shape in relation to each other. That's more important for the incisors— again, the four upper and lower teeth in the front of the mouth. In general, these and the canines—the teeth on either side of the incisors—are rounder than other teeth. Again, it's all based on the individual patient.

I also look at minute details, such as the embrasure, which is the small, v-shaped space where the biting edge of the teeth meet. Starting at the midline of the teeth, the embrasure should get progressively larger between the teeth toward the back of the mouth. I address that during the manicuring process at the end of treatment, which I'll discuss more in chapter 6.

When teeth are crowded, they wear unevenly on the edges. That uneven wear is more apparent after the teeth are straightened. Once teeth are aligned, irregularities and any fractured or broken edges disrupt the pleasing flow of the line along the biting edge of the row of teeth. Correcting these issues is done during manicuring.

The gumline is also an important component of a smile. A gumline that is uneven—for instance, higher on one of the front teeth than the other—is less attractive and can even be distracting. Orthodontics also look at what's known as the "clinical crown," which is how much of the tooth is showing. Sometimes, there's too much gum covering the teeth; sometimes the gums have receded, showing too much of the tooth.

Another issue with the gums is what's known as a "gummy smile." That's when too much gum tissue shows during a smile, or when too little of the teeth show. Typically, younger smiles tend to show more of the gumline, but as a person ages, the gums may recede. That's one reason a gummy smile in a younger person is not always something that needs correction, because it may do so on its own, over time. I'm a prime example of that. When I was a teenager, a lot of my gum tissue showed when I smiled. Today, hardly any of my gum tissue shows.

## The Science of Moving Teeth

My degree in mechanical engineering has helped me immensely as an orthodontist. It has helped me understand the complicated force systems needed to align the teeth. With that education, I learned about forces and vectors, center of rotation, and moment arms—basically the science and mathematics of moving an object.

My educational background also includes a master's degree in dentistry, which I earned during my orthodontics residency. For my master's degree, which required me to research and then present a thesis on a topic, I chose to study the forces applied to teeth that were bonded with a lingual appliance. A lingual appliance, as I mentioned in the introduction, is bonded to the back of the teeth. Today, I combine my engineering education, mathematical analysis of forces, and knowledge of tooth movement to create individualized treatment plans for patients before their appliances are constructed.

There is also a biological science component to understanding how teeth move through bone. Years ago, the classic theory was to apply lots of pressure to the teeth and eventually the teeth would move. But today, we understand more about how teeth move and what makes them move, and we have found that constant, light force is a much better and more efficient way to move teeth.

Teeth live in bone. When a tooth is pushed toward the bone, the bone has different proteins and genes that actually cause the area of the bone in front of the tooth to dissolve, to allow the tooth to move into that space. Then behind the tooth, new bone forms in the area the tooth just vacated. Again, genes and proteins cause that bone growth to occur.

Pushing with too much force interferes with that bone breaking down and the regrowth process, because it cuts off the blood circulation to the area, and doesn't allow the genes and proteins to do their job. That's why today's braces and Invisalign clear aligners, which use lighter forces, are actually able to move teeth more efficiently than systems in the past. Since they are so much more efficient, they allow us to make enough space for all the teeth in the mouth, which can help avoid extractions in many cases.

In order to move teeth, we have to apply certain forces to them. Braces, which attach to teeth, work by pulling teeth into place. Aligners, which are not attached to the teeth, work by pushing teeth into place. Both still apply force and will move teeth in a desired direction, but the challenge for the orthodontist is to figure out how to use the force that's being applied. Again, it all comes down to the training and experience of the professional using the tool, not the tool itself.

## The Technologies

While the best outcomes for your unique smile are the work of the orthodontist guiding treatment, it certainly helps to have some of the latest technologies to accomplish those goals.

In this ever-evolving field, change is a constant. As I write this book, here are some of the latest technologies we use.

**Cone beam computed tomography (CBCT)**. Cone beam computed tomography (CBCT) machines have actually been around for a long time. Doctors have used them to treat patients for many years, and it's only recently that they've been used in orthodontics. The reason orthodontists did not use them much in the past is because they emitted a lot of radiation. But today's machines are vastly improved, exposing patients to a minimal amount of radiation (about as much as an hour in the sun). In my office, I currently use the i-CAT FLX CBCT.

With the CBCT, I can even x-ray underlying structures, which gives me a much better view of the teeth, including any teeth that have yet to erupt. That includes impacted teeth. The images produced by the CBCT help me guide those impacted teeth into the mouth, because I can see where they are in relation to other teeth.

The CBCT also produces images of the jaw joints, which helps me to see whether there are any issues with the TMJ.

I can even see the airway with CBCT images, from the sinuses down to the throat. The CBCT lets me view and measure any constriction in the airway, which is tremendously helpful for determining whether obstructive sleep apnea (OSA) is likely present. It allows me to see, for instance, whether the tonsils or adenoids are potentially causing obstruction of the airway; if so, then I can refer the patient to an ENT for treatment. If it appears there's not enough room for the tongue, then there are orthodontic treatments to help make more room for it to help keep it out of the back of the throat.

*The 3-D scanner we use has been one of the greatest tools that we've brought onboard, because it eliminates the need for impressions that we used to make in order to create a mold of the mouth.*

**3-D scanner (i-Tero Element 2).** The 3-D scanner we use has been one of the greatest tools that we've brought onboard, because it eliminates the need for impressions that we used to make in order to create a mold of the mouth. Taking impressions involved placing a tray of "goop" over the teeth and waiting for it to harden, then creating a model out of plaster that was trimmed and sent off to the lab. It was considered by many to be one of the most unpleasant experiences in orthodontics, or as one of my young patients calls it: "The worst forty-five seconds of my whole life." He and I laughed about his comment when he said it after having an impression, but there was certainly some truth to his statement.

We use the scanner to take images of the teeth, which are then loaded onto a computer to give us a 3-D study model of the mouth. The scanner is basically a video camera on the end of a wand, which is moved around the teeth to create a digital model that then displays on a computer screen. Patients can actually watch their teeth forming in 3-D as we're scanning. By the time the scan is complete, their whole dentition is on-screen. Then, with a single click and a two- or three-minute wait, we can see side-by-side images predicting the patient's teeth before and after treatment. It's a pretty amazing tool and gives the patient a chance to envision what their teeth may look like after they are straightened.

We then use that digital study model to make different appliances such as retainers and expanders. (For a discussion of retainers, see chapter 7.)

We also use the scanner to create the digital model of a patient's teeth before Invisalign treatment. I am able to then manipulate the model of the teeth into the position that is best for that patient, and more importantly, control the sequence of movements in the treatment. That treatment sequence (using a setup by Invisalign known as ClinCheck) is then used to make the series of aligners.

**3-D printer**. The 3-D printer is changing the way orthodontists practice. These are used to print out the model of the patient's teeth at the end of treatment, which is then used to create their retainer.

We have 3-D printers in each office. So now, we can print out the model and make the retainer same day or the next day. We don't always need to deliver the retainers this quickly, but it is nice to have when we need to rush the process.

**Diode laser**. The diode laser is used to help expose teeth that are having trouble erupting. Normally, when a baby tooth comes out, the permanent tooth erupts into the hole left by the baby tooth. But if the tooth is delayed coming in, the tissue in the mouth heals and can prevent the permanent tooth from erupting. The upper canines are notorious for this. By numbing the area and then using the diode laser, I can expose the impacted tooth and put a brace on it that day to bring the impacted tooth into the mouth, reducing treatment time by several months. The diode laser is also used to contour gum tissue to make the gums look more symmetric. This is sometimes done at the end of treatment as part of the finishing touches.

## Accelerated Orthodontics

Orthodontists are always looking for ways to make orthodontic treatment go faster because, in addition to comfort and esthetics, one of the patients' primary concerns is how long treatment will take.

These days, there are technologies designed to make teeth move faster. These innovations take advantage of the role of the genes and proteins in moving teeth.

One of the treatments I use is called micropulse technology. Orthopedic surgeons have long used this technology on bones that wouldn't heal easily. They'd just apply a micropulse, or vibration, to the bone to stimulate the healing process. Often, the bone would then heal without having to involve surgery. Since tooth movement involves a very similar process to the healing process for fractured bones, a couple of devices take advantage of that process to help move teeth a little faster.

One of the devices is known as AcceleDent, the other is the Propel VPro5.

Both of these devices involve the patient biting down onto a mouthpiece for a few minutes a day. The unit vibrates the mouthpiece, which helps to stimulate the bone around the teeth. That stimulation helps speed up the process of the genes and proteins that break down and rebuild bone and are involved in moving teeth.

In the orthodontic community, there's still a split decision on whether micropulse therapy truly works to speed up treatment. Even though more research needs to be done, I've had at least a few cases where it actually seems to do what it's designed to do. For instance, I've had a couple of patients come in to have their teeth straightened before an event five months away. Even though the aligner treatment should have taken twelve months, they used the Propel VPro5 for five minutes every day, and then changed out their aligners every four days, instead of every seven days. Sure enough, it worked. They were able to complete their treatment in less time.

Another way to accelerate tooth movement is with a procedure that actually traumatizes the bone around the teeth. The procedure involves making tiny holes or perforations in the bone around the teeth, which stimulates the proteins and genes and makes the teeth move faster.

I've used the procedure on a couple of patients and it does work, but it is far more invasive. I used it on one adult that had a maxillary (upper) tooth that had been impacted for years. With braces, I was able to get the tooth to erupt through her gum tissue, but couldn't get it to move into place. She agreed to try the perforation procedure and it worked—amazingly, by the following visit, her tooth had moved into place.

Research today is also looking at some other tools, including laser-light technology, to move teeth faster, and even injecting specific genes and proteins around the teeth to help tooth movement. Who knows what's in the future for orthodontics? But one thing is certain: It's an exciting time to be an orthodontist. And for somebody who loves learning, it's a lot of fun to be part of an industry with so many new ways to help patients get the smile they've always imagined.

*It's an exciting time to be an orthodontist.*

# CHAPTER THREE

# THE "TOOLS" I USE
# FOR MOVING TEETH

It's a common misconception that wearing braces or clear aligners such as Invisalign is what straightens teeth. But to repeat my earlier message, the outcome of treatment is not determined by the braces, Invisalign, auxiliary appliances, or any other tools that are used to move teeth. What makes a difference in outcomes for any patient is the expertise of the orthodontist guiding treatment. That's why experience is key when choosing an orthodontist.

Most problems in the mouth can be corrected. The degree to which they can be corrected often comes down to how complex the treatment is, which can affect the costs. For instance, redirecting jaw growth and development in children is a much more affordable treatment than orthognathic (jaw) surgery in adults. That's why we recommend early treatment for patients that have severe problems. At age seven, we can create space in a young child's jaw to prevent severe crowding that can cause problems in the future. Taking advantage of a still-developing jaw in a child is also one of the best ways to deal with some types of airway issues that are being seen in so many adults these days. I'll talk more about these and other issues specific to children and youth in the next chapter.

## Types of Bites

The underlying goal of all orthodontic treatment is to create the best occlusion, or best bite, for each individual. Webster's Dictionary defines malocclusion as "an abnormality in the coming together of teeth." What that basically means is that the teeth don't meet as they should during a bite. A good bite is the foundation for long-term oral and overall health.

The positioning of the teeth and their support of the lips is also a measure of a good outcome with orthodontics. If the teeth are too far forward, the lips may appear abnormally full—the patient may not even be able to close their lips properly. Conversely, if the teeth are too far back and the lips are under-supported, they look thin and wrinkled. That's what makes a face look older.

*Correcting a bite has both esthetic and functional purposes.*

So, correcting a bite has both esthetic and functional purposes.

There are three different classes of occlusions:

- Class I is a good bite. It's when the upper and lower teeth come together well during a bite, and they function as they are supposed to.

- Class II is a malocclusion, or bad bite. It's where all the upper teeth are more forward than they should be in relation to the lower teeth.

- Class III is a malocclusion, or bad bite. It's where the lower teeth are more forward than they should be in the relation to the upper teeth.

These classes include several types of bites that orthodontics can correct.

**Underbite**. An underbite is when the lower teeth jut out farther than the upper teeth. An underbite can lead to serious issues such as abnormal teeth wear, poor chewing, and an unsightly smile. An underbite can be caused by abnormal jaw growth, or by improper tooth position.

**Crossbite**. This malocclusion occurs when the upper teeth are inside the lower teeth during a bite. This forces patients to move their lower jaw forward or to the side in order to close their mouth, which is an improper use of the lower jaw, and can sometimes cause facial asymmetry.

Crossbites can be anterior, which means in the front teeth, or posterior, which means in the back teeth. Or, there can be both anterior and posterior crossbites.

Crossbites lead to abnormal tooth wear, direct biting trauma to the teeth, and serious gum problems where the teeth are literally forced out of the gums, if the crossbite is severe enough.

Crossbites are one reason the American Association of Orthodontics recommends that every child be screened by age seven, because this particular bite is so much easier to correct at a younger age than as an adult. It is much easier to correct at age seven, eight, or nine. As an adult, sometimes the only way to correct a crossbite is with jaw surgery.

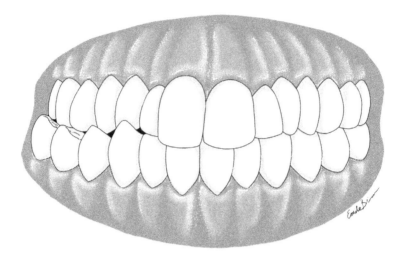

*Posterior Crossbite*

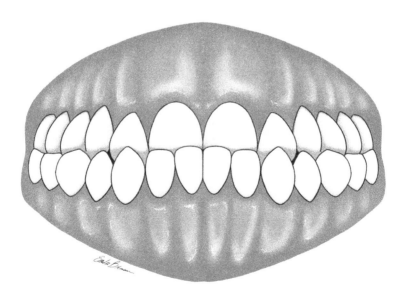

*Anterior Crossbite*

**Overjet (or upper front teeth protrusion)**. This bite is characterized by the upper teeth extending too far forward, or the lower teeth not extending far enough forward. Sometimes, an overjet is caused by the position of the teeth, sometimes it is the position of the jaws.

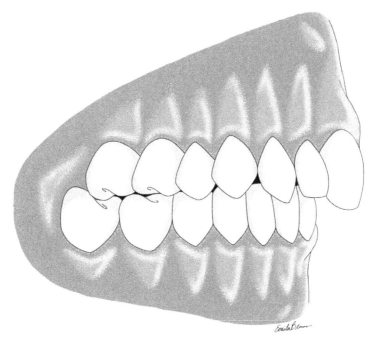

*Excessive Overjet*

I've seen damage to teeth quite often in children with a large overjet or protruding teeth. The child will fall or hit something with their mouth, causing a fracture of a front tooth or teeth. Fractures or even losing a tooth or teeth altogether is pretty common when someone has a severe overjet.

An overjet is often mistakenly termed an overbite, which is the type of bite I'll discuss next. But there is a difference between the two—again, an overjet is when the upper front teeth protrude forward.

**Overbite (or deep bite).** In an overbite, the upper front teeth overlap the lower front teeth, concealing the lower front teeth when a smile is viewed from the front. In a good bite, the upper teeth should only overlap the lower front teeth by about 20 percent. A deep overbite, where the lower teeth are completely concealed by the upper front teeth, can sometimes cause the lower front teeth to actually bite into the roof of the mouth. Other problems that are often associated with an overbite include excessive wear on the front teeth, lips that protrude too far forward, and a "gummy" smile, where too much of the gum tissue shows during a smile.

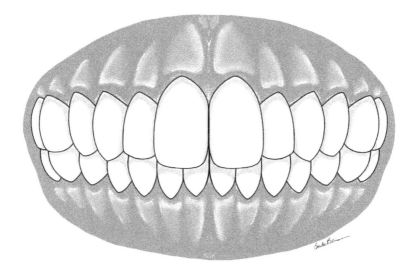

*Excessive Overbite*

**Crowding or crooked teeth.** Crowding occurs when there is not enough room for the teeth to erupt during development. Crowding creates crooked teeth, which is one of the most common reasons for people to seek orthodontic treatment. Not only is crowding unattractive, but crowded teeth that overlap can harbor bacterial plaque, increasing the risk for tooth decay and gum disease, because it's so much more difficult to keep them clean. And, as I mentioned in chapter 1, dental decay and gum disease can lead to heart disease, diabetes, and other serious health issues.

Crowded or crooked teeth are also a symptom of a jaw that is too narrow for the tongue to rest comfortably in, which can lead to obstructive sleep apnea (OSA). In the past, it was common to extract teeth to make more room for all the remaining teeth to grow in. But today, there are better ways to deal with crowding. Specifically, we can direct jaw growth to get a broader smile or broader jaw. That can, in turn, help prevent or alleviate OSA (more about obstructive sleep apnea in chapters 5 and 6).

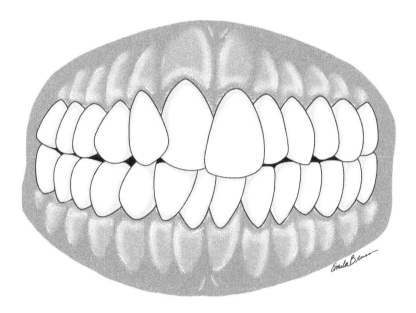

*Crowding*

**Spacing**. Another common reason for patients to seek orthodontic treatment is the spaces or gaps between their teeth. Although not generally a serious health problem, large gaps between teeth can ruin an otherwise beautiful smile. Although some celebrities are known for the gap in between their two front teeth, most patients that I see with gaps in their teeth are very self-conscious about them. I had gaps in my teeth as a youth, which was one of the reasons I wanted braces.

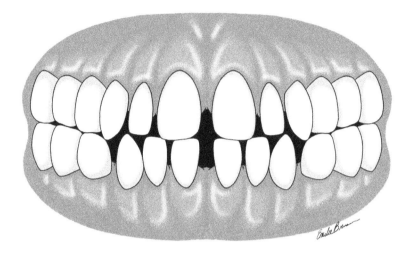

*Spacing*

**Open bite**. In an open bite, the front teeth don't meet. This bite can be caused by the way the jaw grew during development. When the lower jaw grows into a more downward position, it can cause an open bite because the teeth just can't grow up far enough to meet together. When we take an x-ray of the side of the head, we measure the angles of the jaws. If the patient's lower jaw really seems to tilt down and they have a long lower face, then the front teeth have a longer way to grow as they try to erupt to come together. That lets us know we're looking at a potential problem with development.

Open bite can also be the result of a tongue thrust, where the tongue chronically pushes between the upper and lower front teeth. If a person has enlarged adenoids or tonsils, they can't breathe through their nose correctly, so they breathe through their mouth, which causes them to position their tongue forward. If a patient comes to me with an open bite, I want to determine what's causing it, if possible, and not just correct it, because there are different ways to correct an open bite, depending on the cause. If the cause is their tonsils or adenoids, then I refer them to an ENT.

An open bite can also be caused by a habit, like thumb-sucking. We have solutions to resolve these habits early on, and I'll talk about them later in the chapter.

Early evaluation and intervention are essential in correcting an open bite. Left untreated, an open bite can lead to excessive wear on the back teeth because all of the biting forces are only on the back teeth. I've actually seen open bite cause the loss of the back teeth, because they're just so traumatized by taking on all the forces of chewing.

While the problem is more prominently seen in children, I see it in adults, too. The good news is that Invisalign clear aligners can often be used to correct open bites more successfully than braces.

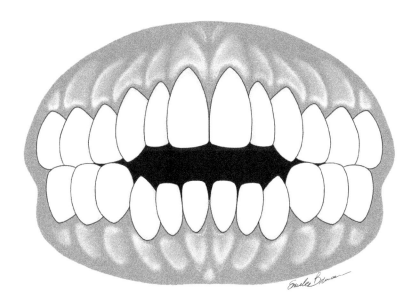

*Open Bite*

**Mismatched dental midlines**. A mismatched midline is when the upper and lower front teeth don't meet in the middle. If the upper midline is off to one side or another, of course, it really shows in a photograph. However, the midline may be off because of a tooth that is too small on one side of the mouth. A mismatched midline is very easy to correct before all the patient's teeth have erupted, but once all the teeth have erupted, it's much more difficult to align the midlines. That's why correcting a midline in an adult can sometimes be a difficult treatment to undergo.

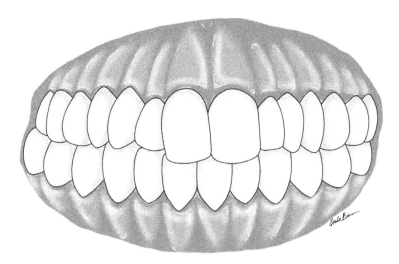

*Mismatched Dental Midlines*

**Abnormal eruptions**. Abnormal eruptions, also known as ectopic eruptions, are teeth that erupt out of position. An abnormal eruption can occur almost anywhere in the mouth—in the roof of the mouth or simply in the wrong place compared to other teeth. Abnormal eruptions include impacted teeth, or teeth that have the potential to impact, which is something I see every day.

Abnormal eruptions are much easier to correct in young people than in adults. It's easier to move teeth out of the way in a young person's mouth to make room for teeth that are coming in. At a young age, we can also redirect jaw growth much more easily. Or, we may even remove a baby tooth rather than wait until it impacts, because once it's impacted, then it may need the attention of an oral surgeon.

## Tools for Moving Teeth

The tools used for moving teeth depend on the patient's individual situation. For instance, one of the big advantages of Invisalign clear aligners is that they can correct many open bites more effectively than braces. Deep bites, on the other hand, are more easily corrected with braces.

Determining which tool is best is where the experience and expertise of the orthodontist have the greatest impact. Here are the tools I use most, depending on the corrections needed.

**Braces**. Today's braces look very similar to braces of the past, but they are more effective and efficient at moving teeth. Braces are composed of brackets bonded or glued to the teeth accompanied by a wire that is inserted into the brackets.

In the past, the wire was held in place with a rubber band or wire. The braces I use today hold the wire in place with a little door on the bracket that closes down over the wire. This type of bracket, known as self-ligating, has been in use for some time. Self-ligating refers to the door that closes down over the wire, allowing it to ligate or tie itself in. With self-ligating braces, there is a lot less friction and binding of the wire in the brackets, which allows it to move more freely to straighten the teeth.

When I first heard about self-ligating brackets, I thought they couldn't make that much difference. Then, after trying them, it was obvious that the bracket made a huge difference. Since I began using the self-ligating system, I've seen it do amazing things.

The wires themselves are also different today. They used to only be available in stainless steel, which is a fairly rigid material. These days, the initial wire put on the teeth is much more flexible. The wire was made for the space industry, to be used as satellite antennae. It was designed to be very pliable when cold, allowing it to be coiled up for storage during flight. Then, once the satellite was in space, the wire was warmed up by the sun, causing it to uncoil.

We use the same technology with our orthodontic wires. They are kept in a refrigerator until ready for use. When they are placed in the mouth, they warm up. The wires have "memory," which is key to moving the teeth. Once the wire warms up in the mouth, it returns to its original shape, and pulls the teeth along with it.

Treatment begins with that very light, flexible, memory wire. Then, once the teeth are straightened, the memory wire is removed and replaced with more rigid stainless-steel wire. That stronger, more rigid wire is needed to move the teeth into the final form.

Braces come in traditional metal or clear ceramic. Some adult patients who do not choose Invisalign as a treatment option elect for clear ceramic. However, more and more people are realizing the many advantages in using Invisalign treatment.

Many younger patients want metal braces because they use bands, known as alastics, that come in a multitude of colors. Although the metal braces I use today don't require bands, patients that want them are given a choice of colors. But it is becoming much more common for patients at all ages to choose Invisalign over metal braces because there is less discomfort, less risk of white spots or cavities, no restrictions on eating, and teeth are easier to clean because the aligners are removable.

## Keep Your New Smile Healthy

Patients that choose to wear braces must take extra care with their oral hygiene every day to ensure the healthiest smile—their best smile. Patients are supplied with brushing and flossing kits, along with instructions, once their braces are placed. Here are the guidelines patients must follow to ensure the best brushing and flossing around braces:

- Use a soft, hand-held, micro-bristle brush to clean the hard-to-reach tiny crevices in the brackets or in between teeth, where food particles and bacteria can get caught. A hard-bristle brush can actually traumatize the gum tissue and cause it to recede.

- When brushing, also clean slightly underneath and along the gumline to massage the gums.

- Use a fluoride toothpaste to help restore essential vitamins and minerals that make teeth stronger and more resistant to decay.

- Angle the bristles of the brush at forty-five degrees to the gumline. Move the brush in tiny circles around teeth and gums. Don't scrub too hard to avoid damaging your gums.

- Brush along the front, back, and chewing surfaces until all of your teeth have been cleaned.

- Flossing with braces can be a challenge, due to the wires between the teeth. I used to time myself, and it took eleven minutes to floss. A floss threader is a small device that helps slide the floss underneath the arch wire. There are also air flossers available, which use a powerful stream of air to remove debris between teeth.

- Floss thoroughly in between all gaps in the teeth, both above and below the wire.

- Other tools that work well to remove debris include a proxy brush, which is a very small toothbrush that looks like a tiny Christmas tree on the end of a wire. It can easily fit in between braces, the arch wire, and the spaces between teeth. Water picks, which clean teeth using a thin, powerful stream of water, are good auxiliary tools to use, but should not replace brushing and flossing.

- It's recommended to brush after every meal, which isn't always easy to do at school or at work. At minimum, brush before bedtime and upon waking in the morning.

- Flossing should follow brushing, which again, isn't always easy to do. At minimum, floss once a day, ideally before bedtime.

## Eating with Braces

Certain foods can create problems with braces. Hard, crunchy, or very chewy foods can break or damage wires and brackets. Sticky foods can get caught between brackets and wires. Nail biting, pencil and pen chewing, and chewing on foreign objects can break braces. Here are some food guidelines when wearing braces.

- Avoid sticky foods, such as taffy, caramels, licorice, toffee, bubble gum, Starburst, Tootsie Rolls, and Sugar Daddies. Sugarless gum is okay to chew, since it is softer and won't damage brackets, and there is no sugar to cause decay or damage teeth.

- Avoid hard foods such as ice, nuts, crispy taco shells, crusty breads, pretzels, popcorn, and Jolly Ranchers. Ice can actually make brackets and wires flex and change shape, which can cause them to loosen and break. Popcorn has husks that can get caught underneath the gums, causing infection and pain.

- Cut into bite-size pieces, and chew with the back teeth, foods such as apples, raw carrots, bagels, pizza, chips, and corn on the cob (cut the corn from the cob).

- Minimize sugary foods such as cake, ice cream, cookies, pie, and candy. Sugary foods can cause tooth decay. Sugar left on the teeth around brackets can cause permanent scarring (white spots).

- Avoid carbonated drinks, sodas, and drinks that contain sugar, as much as possible.

## What Counts as an Orthodontic Emergency?

While orthodontic emergencies are extremely rare, they can significantly disrupt treatment. With all my years of experience and learning when to apply braces, combined with today's improved technologies, we're now able to avoid most emergencies that patients might have.

Still, emergencies do occur, in different levels of severity. But sometimes, what can seem like a dire situation can be treated at home, followed by an in-office appointment.

For instance, the main minor emergencies we see involve a loose or broken bracket, band, or wire; an archwire that is poking the inside of the cheek; general discomfort; or the feeling that teeth are loose. Loose or broken brackets, bands, or wires are typically caused by eating hard or sticky foods. If any of these components become dislodged, give us a call at the office to set up an appointment, and then hold onto the component until we can place it back on the teeth. An archwire poking a cheek can cause irritation, which can be remedied by moving the wire with a pencil eraser, tweezers, or Q-tip, or by covering the end of the wire with orthodontic wax until your appointment. For general discomfort or a feeling of loose teeth, an over-the-counter pain reliever, salt water rinse, or warm compress can often provide relief.

Major emergencies, on the other hand, include trauma or injury to the teeth, face, or mouth; infection or swelling in the mouth or gums; and severe discomfort. With any of these, contact the office immediately. In the case of trauma—such as colliding with someone else on an athletic field—a visit to the emergency room may be in order. Once the problem is addressed there, then a visit to the office is likely in order to repair any damage to the braces.

**Invisalign (clear aligners).** As I stated earlier, many patients want to avoid all the extra care and restrictions that come with wearing braces. An alternative to braces is customized clear aligners, plastic trays that fit very nicely over the teeth. Right now, Invisalign is the premier provider of clear aligners on the market. Invisalign aligners are made of a unique, patented, dual-layer plastic called SmartTrack. It's the most effective material being used today for aligning teeth.

Invisalign has a unique process that pushes teeth into place, as opposed to pulling teeth, like braces do. These custom aligners are designed specifically for each tooth's unique movement. Invisalign is for people that don't want braces showing during treatment, and for whom speaking clearly is important (since lingual braces, those that bond to the back of the teeth, can cause speaking problems for some people).

Teen athletes and band musicians like Invisalign because the aligners reduce the risk of trauma from impact during play or while playing an instrument. High school seniors, especially, like Invisalign because they don't show in senior pictures and prom photos. Athletes also like Invisalign because adjustments are only required once every twelve weeks, so there is less chance of missing a practice and being left out of a game as a result. Since game seasons are typically about three months long, we can schedule visits before and after.

Invisalign is also a better choice for college-age individuals, especially if their school is in a neighboring city. Should a bracket come loose with traditional braces, it can be difficult to come in for a repair. With Invisalign, if an aligner is lost, the patient usually just moves up to the next aligner in the series. Again, the flexible visit schedule with Invisalign makes orthodontic treatment much more viable for these patients.

Invisalign has become such a key player in orthodontics that the next chapter covers it in great detail.

**Auxiliary appliances**. There are many different types of auxiliary appliances available to help move teeth and jaws during treatment. Here are the most common ones that I use, depending on the patient's situation:

- **Expanders** are used to widen the upper palate in young patients. I most often use a "quad helix," which applies gentle force that reshapes the jaw over about a six- to eight-month period. I usually don't use the more common rapid palatal expander, (that makes the movements in a much shorter time period) because that appliance tends to be more painful.

- **Elastics (rubber bands) and the Herbst appliance**. Elastics, or rubber bands, attach the upper to the lower braces on the sides of the mouth. These are used to help correct how the upper and lower teeth meet (occlusion), and must be changed out by the patient throughout treatment.

  Today, I also use what's known as a Herbst appliance for specific corrections, such as an overbite or deficient lower jaw growth. In fact, if the Herbst appliance had existed when I was young and needed my overbite corrected, the orthognathic surgery I had when I finished dental school could have been avoided.

  A Herbst appliance is a stainless-steel bar that, like the rubber bands, connects to the braces on the upper and lower teeth on the side of the mouth and helps guide growth of the jaw. Unlike rubber bands, however, patients cannot remove the Herbst appliance. However, it only works while a jaw is still developing, so it's something that must be done at an earlier age—typically into the early teens at the latest.

Elastics and the Herbst appliance take the place of headgear, which is a device connected to the braces but worn outside the mouth. Headgear was worn in the past to guide jaw development. Today, I joke with patients that it's an option if they don't wear their rubber bands as prescribed.

As I write this book, a couple of the newest options available for guiding jaw development are "Invisalign First" and "Invisalign Teen." These clear aligners can now perform many of the desired corrections previously only possible with fixed appliances, such as a Herbst appliance or a quad helix.

- **Space maintainers** are used often in my practice. These help hold space open when baby teeth have fallen out or when a child has lost their baby teeth very early. Space maintainers prevent the adjacent permanent teeth from moving into the space left by the baby teeth, while leaving enough space open for other teeth to erupt.

- **Habit appliances** are designed to correct bad habits that could lead to issues with oral development, which may require extensive treatment to correct. The two main habits include thumb-sucking and tongue thrust. With thumb-sucking, pressure from the thumb is consistently being exerted onto the developing teeth and jaw bone. With tongue thrusting, the tongue is continually pushing forward between the upper and lower front teeth. Either can lead to deformation or slowed growth of the bone, as well as severely misaligned teeth that flare out towards the lips and create an open bite. A habit appliance can correct these problems by providing a "block" to keep the thumb out of the mouth or to keep the tongue from pushing between the teeth. A tongue thrust habit must be corrected by age eight or nine or it will become so ingrained that it can never be properly corrected with orthodontics alone—it will require additional help from a speech-language therapist or other specialists.

## Partner Providers

To provide patients comprehensive treatment, I often work with dentists and other specialists.

**General dentists** offer a number of services that complement orthodontics. They maintain the health of the dentition by providing care during regular visits, checkups, and cleaning appointments. General dentists (or family dentists) also provide a multitude of services such as placing crowns on teeth to protect them or placing crowns on implants. They also place bridges for missing teeth and provide dental whitening to improve the shade of teeth. Many dentists also place veneers to improve the appearance of teeth.

**Oral surgeons** often help expose teeth that are impacted in the bone and apply a chain to the tooth that is used by the orthodontist to guide the impacted tooth into the mouth. Oral surgeons also place implants that later receive crowns to replace missing teeth, and they perform orthognathic surgery (jaw surgery). Oral surgeons also help us with those pesky wisdom teeth that often cause crowding as they attempt to erupt.

**Periodontists** are crucial for treating patients who develop gum disease, which can lead to tooth loss. They can also contour the gum tissue when it has overgrown over the teeth. Periodontists can also help with gum tissue that has overgrown, causing a gap between teeth. That tissue, known as the frenum, connects the upper lip to the upper gum. A periodontist can clip that tissue, and then an orthodontist can close the gap with braces.

**Pediatric dentists** perform many of the functions general dentists provide, but with a special emphasis on treating children. For instance, a pediatric dentist can help with a child that has a special orthodontic issue, such as a baby tooth that needs to be removed to allow a permanent tooth come in. We send such cases to a pediatric dentist, because the procedures they perform are less traumatizing for the patient.

**Ear, nose, and throat specialists (ENTs)** can remove tonsils and adenoids if imaging from the CBCT x-ray machine reveals that a patient has a constricted airway in the back of the throat. Removing tonsils and adenoids can help open the patient's airway and potentially prevent OSA.

Now let's take a look at the orthodontic "tool" that is taking the lead in orthodontic treatment.

# CHAPTER FOUR

# INVISALIGN CLEAR ALIGNER THERAPY—A NEW WORLD OF ORTHODONTICS

Clear aligner therapy is revolutionizing the profession of orthodontics. It's opening up a whole new world for many people who strongly desire to straighten their teeth and get their best smile, but really don't want traditional braces.

*Clear aligner therapy is revolutionizing the profession of orthodontics.*

When Invisalign first hit the market in 1998, the treatment was very limited in what it could accomplish. Mild crowding and mild spacing issues—those were about the only problems that Invisalign could be used for when it first came out.

Today, with the advances in Invisalign as a digital technology, many, many more patients can be treated and obtain superb results.

And the types of cases we can treat successfully are increasing almost daily.

As I write this book, I am an Invisalign patient myself. When I created my own Invisalign treatment plan, my teeth were still straight from wearing braces more than twenty years ago (because I've worn my retainers). But I wanted a broader smile and also wanted to see what my patients were experiencing with Invisalign.

I've found that I'm able to speak very well while wearing my aligners. To me, there is a big difference in the comfort between braces and Invisalign. With Invisalign, there is very little soreness and it is much easier to keep my teeth clean, because I can remove the aligners to brush and floss. I also remove them while eating, so there are no restrictions on my diet, as would be the case if I had braces. Invisalign is just a whole lot easier to work into my lifestyle. I change the aligners once a week per my treatment plan, and I can already tell a big difference in my smile.

## What Is Clear Aligner Treatment?

- Invisalign is a brand of clear aligner treatment that is being used more and more these days to straighten teeth. Having been engaged in clear aligner therapy since 1998, the company now has more experience in moving teeth faster and better. It has invested millions of dollars in research over the years to continually improve how its aligners work. There are other brands on the market, but Invisalign is currently the brand of choice in my practice.

- Instead of straightening teeth through a system of brackets and wires like traditional braces, Invisalign uses special aligners that are made from a durable, translucent plastic.

The aligners are designed to fit over the teeth like a shell, and are practically invisible when worn. When the aligners are placed on the teeth, they apply small amounts of pressure to the teeth and jaws to make the corrections determined by the orthodontist. Unlike braces that pull teeth into place, Invisalign aligners push on teeth to move them into their new positions.

To create the aligners, the orthodontist takes a mold or digital scan of the upper and lower teeth and sends it along with x-rays and photos to the Invisalign lab. With the digital model of the teeth, Invisalign technicians use a highly-sophisticated CAD/CAM system to create the series of aligners for patients. Before the aligners are made, however, the technicians use the digital model to create what is known as a setup (called a ClinCheck), which places the teeth into the position the technicians determine the teeth will move. That ClinCheck is sent back to the orthodontist for approval.

All of this is done digitally, via the internet. It's an amazing advancement in orthodontics and represents one of the reasons that Invisalign is currently the industry leader.

Still, technicians are not orthodontists. They follow certain guidelines as they create the setup, but often the movements pre-scribed are not ideal, or even feasible. They have not undergone the training that an orthodontist has in order to understand the parameters of tooth movement. As the treating orthodontist, I must review the setup they create, and make changes to optimize the treatment. It's not uncommon for me to modify the treatment plan multiple times before finally approving it.

As I mentioned in chapter 2, I earned a master's degree in dentistry while I was going to orthodontic residency, and part of that included researching how forces applied to teeth cause them to move.

Interestingly, the makers of Invisalign are using the same sciences that I learned in school to analyze the forces needed with clear aligner therapy. They use very sophisticated machines and computers to study the complex forces required for tooth movement using aligners.

## Caring for Invisalign

Aligners are most effective when worn twenty-two hours a day. Most of my treatment plans allow the patient to switch out their aligners weekly, moving to the next aligner in the series. If they lose an aligner or their pet takes a liking to it (dogs love to chew on plastic aligners), most of the time, the patient can move up to the next aligner in the series and wear it for two weeks, instead of one. That way, the missing aligner doesn't have to be replaced. However, if for some reason the next aligner doesn't fit, then we can reorder a replacement aligner from Invisalign. During treatment, up to six aligners can be replaced at no additional charge.

With Invisalign, visits for adjustments take place approximately every twelve weeks. That means, in between those visits, it's up to you, the patient, to wear your aligners as recommended and switch them out to the next in the series in order to ensure teeth move as planned. Here are some instructions we give to patients with Invisalign.

- My team will give you instructions on how to insert the aligners to make them work most effectively. They will show you how to fully seat them using "chewies," and how to push the aligners over the attachments (called "massaging" the attachments).

- Wear the aligners as instructed and take them out only for eating and brushing. When removing them to eat or brush, place them in the case that is provided to avoid losing or damaging the aligner by mislaying it, tossing it out with a napkin from your meal, breaking it by trying to store it in a pocket, or leaving it where the dog can get at it.

- You can drink with the aligners in, as even hot liquids will not harm them, but it is a good idea to rinse out any liquids containing sugar.

- Some soreness is expected, as teeth will start moving right away. Advil or Tylenol should provide adequate pain relief.

- When removing the aligners to brush your teeth, brush the aligners with your toothbrush and either soap or toothpaste. It is not recommended to soak them in retainer or denture cleanser.

- Please keep all of your old aligners in a safe place, as you may need to go back to a previous aligner.

## Advantages of Invisalign

Many patients are given the choice of braces or Invisalign. In addition to being nearly invisible, here are some of the reasons a patient might choose Invisalign:

- **Removable for cleaning teeth.** The aligners are not bonded to the teeth, so they are easy to remove for brushing and flossing. That makes it easier to have good oral hygiene throughout treatment.

- **Removable for eating.** Since the aligners can be removed, they are taken out for meals. That means there is no special diet required throughout treatment.

- **Less soreness.** The material used for the aligners is soft and flexible, which is less irritating on the soft tissues of the mouth than metal braces. The therapy also uses light forces to move teeth, which is a more comfortable type of movement.

- **Protection for teeth-grinding.** For patients that have a habit of grinding or clenching their teeth, clear aligners can function as thin nightguards that protect the teeth from excessive wear, and often help relieve jaw joint issues (TMJ).

- **Doesn't interfere with playing musical instruments.** Braces can be a troublesome issue for patients playing certain instruments, so Invisalign is a great option for them.

- **No worry of trauma during activities.** Traditional braces are a concern for athletes, cheerleaders, and people involved in activities during which they might experience an impact to the mouth. Such an impact could cause injury to their lips and teeth. Patients can remove Invisalign while participating in these activities, or just leave them in, without the worry of trauma.

- **Now available for all ages.** Invisalign initially was only available for adults. But now teenagers and even younger patients can be treated with Invisalign. Early and adolescent treatment will be discussed in the next chapter, and often Invisalign can be used to perform those treatments.

Since Invisalign is able to treat so many more cases today, the choice to have clear aligner therapy or Invisalign often comes down to a personal preference and depends on a patient's lifestyle. For that reason, I don't charge differently for braces or Invisalign. The fee is the same because I want the patient to get what they want, without worrying about additional cost.

## Attachments, Refinements, Interproximal Reduction

Three components of Invisalign treatment make all the difference with Invisalign: attachments, refinements, and interproximal reduction.

**Attachments**. Attachments are really what make Invisalign work. Attachments are clear-colored bumps that are bonded directly to the teeth. Each attachment is specifically designed to provide the necessary grip to help the aligners push on the teeth to move them in the desired direction. The attachments are made of a unique material that is easy to apply to the teeth, doesn't stain, and is easy to remove. They are attached at the beginning of the treatment and removed at the end of the treatment.

Invisalign has developed many unique attachment shapes designed for specific tooth movements. However, I often change the attachments based on what I know is most crucial for the success of the whole treatment, not just for movement of that particular tooth.

During treatment, teeth are not usually moved just one way. They might need to be extruded, they might need to be rotated, or the roots might need to be tipped. Different attachments are designed for different movements; one attachment usually won't do everything that's needed during treatment. That's where refinement comes in.

**Refinements**. The first set of aligners is typically used to make the most difficult moves first. After those movements are completed, then we do what's known as a refinement. That involves taking another scan, ordering another set of aligners, and then, when they arrive, removing the attachments as needed and placing new ones to finish up the case. The refinement happens when treatment is about 80 percent complete. Currently, Invisalign will create up to four sets of aligners at no additional charge to complete treatment, but that many sets are rarely needed. Usually, it takes two, sometimes three sets.

**Interproximal Reduction (IPR)**. Quite often with Invisalign I perform what's known as interproximal reduction (IPR). Sometimes I do this procedure with braces, but it's more common with Invisalign.

IPR is a process that involves mechanically removing small amounts of tooth enamel in between the teeth to create room for straightening them. The keyword there is "small," usually only around .2 to .3 millimeters, and those spaces are closed as treatment progresses. IPR is a safe, quick, and painless procedure.

## The Difference Experience Makes

As I mentioned earlier, Invisalign's lab technicians understand how to create the clear aligners according to a plan. But they don't really understand how teeth move; they just go by the guidelines Invisalign gives them to straighten the teeth. It's up to the orthodontist to determine whether the movements the aligners will make are actually feasible.

Although some general dentists use Invisalign to straighten teeth, most have limited knowledge on how it can really be used to obtain the best result. Orthodontists study how teeth move, and then they go into practice where they spend all day, year after year, moving teeth. General dentists have an extremely important role in oral health, partnering with orthodontists to provide care. While an orthodontist is, in fact, a dentist, he or she has spent years in training and practice beyond dental school specializing in the art and science of moving teeth.

A general dentist usually does not have the experience to understand the intricate movements involved, and so will accept the lab tech's first suggestion. Often, the teeth do not move as the lab projected, so the treatment falls far short of goals.

When it comes to do-it-yourself options that are advertised on television and available online, the situation's even worse because there is no dentist overseeing the work at all. These do-it-yourself options involve getting a scan or impression of the teeth, then aligners are manufactured and mailed out for the patient to use on their own—with no supervision. No attachments or refinements are used, which greatly reduces the aligners' ability to straighten the teeth, much less provide the patient's best smile. I just recently saw a patient who had severe root damage as a result of one of these do-it-yourself treatments.

As you can tell by what I've been discussing in the book so far, orthodontic treatments vary from patient to patient. But age and growth and development do somewhat dictate the types of treatment we're able to offer. In the next chapter, I'll explain the types of treatment for the youngest patients and adolescents, and then, in chapter 6, I'll talk about the different treatments for adults.

CHAPTER FIVE

# DIFFERENT TREATMENTS AT EVERY AGE—EARLY AND ADOLESCENT TREATMENT

Orthodontic treatment differs to some extent, depending on the age of the patient. Treatment can be provided to patients at any age, but there are distinct differences and challenges in treating patients at different age groups. My goal is to provide each patient with the most appropriate treatment at the most appropriate time.

## Early Treatment

The American Association of Orthodontics recommends that every child be screened by age seven. Some of the recommended reasons are so the orthodontist can spot problems with jaw growth and emerging permanent teeth while baby teeth are still present in the mouth.

There are some conditions that are much easier to treat if they're caught at an early age, when a child's natural growth processes can aid treatment. That's because the orthodontist can create space in a young child's jaws to prevent severe crowding or impactions, and take advantage of rapid facial growth to allow the jaw to grow into a more normal position.

*The American Association of Orthodontics recommends that every child be screened by age seven.*

The goals of early treatment are to align the jaws and to alleviate problems that are very difficult to treat later on. Early treatment can also make future treatment the patient may undergo as an adolescent much easier while producing better results. Many patients, however, do not need early treatment, and if so, they are monitored every six to twelve months while more tooth eruption and facial growth occurs.

There are a number of issues that early treatment can correct. Here are the ones that are most commonly seen in young children:

**Protruding teeth** can be damaged or cause self-image issues. Children often present with protruding upper incisors. In fact, many of the young patients I see at age seven or eight have already had a front tooth fractured because they fell and struck it. Sometimes, we even correct protruding teeth to prevent a social issue. Children with protruding teeth often get bullied in school just because of the look of their teeth.

**Impacted teeth**. This is a very common problem that may be prevented with early treatment. At a very young age, it's much easier to make room for permanent teeth to erupt, and avoid oral surgery later as an adult.

Basically, there are three main ways to deal with an impaction, depending on the problem. The first is to deal with the roots of the teeth. When I take a CBCT scan of a young child, I look at whether the roots of the already erupted teeth are "blocking" the eruption of a permanent tooth trying to come in. Sometimes, the roots of the teeth (under the gum) will tip in, instead of remaining upright. If so, I use Invisalign or braces to move the roots out of the way. Another way is to expand the mouth to make enough room for the impacted tooth. Finally, if baby teeth are in the way of the permanent teeth and potentially going to cause an impaction, then sometimes the baby teeth are extracted early to make a path for the eruption of permanent teeth.

If I don't see a child at an early age, and they are dealing with an impacted tooth as an adolescent, then it may mean using the diode laser (see chapter 2) to expose the tooth just under the tissue, or it may require referring them to an oral surgeon, if the tooth is impacted in the bone. The oral surgeon will go in under the tissue, expose the tooth, and then attach a brace to the tooth along with a small gold chain. That chain is then attached to the brackets to guide the tooth into place. Today, impacted teeth can even be guided into the mouth using Invisalign.

**Early loss of baby teeth (primary teeth).** Sometimes a baby tooth has to be extracted because it has a cavity or a fracture. Rarer, but still a problem, is when a permanent tooth comes in and pushes out two baby teeth. When either of these instances occurs, the adjacent permanent teeth can move into the space and block other permanent teeth from coming in. Preventing this problem involves using an appliance known as a space maintainer to hold the space open until the permanent tooth erupts.

**Severe crowding**, corrected early, can possibly eliminate the need to extract permanent teeth at a later date, and possibly avoid oral surgery to retrieve impacted teeth.

At an early age, palatal expansion is often accomplished with an appliance or Invisalign to alleviate severe crowding when the mouth is too small.

**Severe crossbite**. A severe crossbite is most easily corrected when a child is young.

A crossbite is when the upper teeth tip in and are inside the lower teeth during a bite. An anterior crossbite, or a crossbite in the front teeth, can actually make the lower jaw position more forward than it needs to be, causing it to grow into an underbite. A posterior crossbite, which is in the back of the mouth, is a sign that the mouth is not growing wide enough. Palatal expansion is often used to correct a posterior crossbite.

Again, teeth are easier to move in young patients, around ages seven to nine, so it's easier to get more width and proper shape out of a mouth that's still in the developmental stages. But even by the time a child reaches adolescence, most of the facial growth is already complete, making these movements more difficult to accomplish.

**Missing teeth**. As I mentioned, when a patient has a missing tooth or teeth, the space may be held open to allow for permanent teeth to erupt. But a lot of factors actually come into play when deciding what to do with a missing tooth or teeth in the mouth, and many of these decisions are made when the patient is an adolescent. I'll discuss this more under the treatment for adolescents section in this chapter.

**Severe underbite** is often caused by the lower jaw growing faster than the upper jaw. A severe underbite is apparent when the lower teeth appear in front of the upper teeth. Often, an underbite can be corrected at an early age by tipping the upper teeth forward and the lower teeth back. Most of the time, those movements help the jaws develop at the same rate, creating a proper bite. However, in some patients, only so much movement is possible. At that point, we also look at other options—such as extracting lower teeth to allow the lower incisors to be moved back, or orthognathic (jaw) surgery.

**Bad habits** such as thumb-sucking, tongue thrusting, and mouth-breathing are common in young children. As I explained in chapter 3, these can cause an open bite. In addition to being unsightly and dysfunctional, left untreated, an open bite can cause excessive wear on the back teeth, even to the point of loss of the back teeth.

As I mentioned earlier, thumb-sucking and tongue thrust can be corrected with habit appliances are essentially "cages" that block the thumb from being inserted the mouth or prevent the tongue from constantly pushing between the upper and lower front teeth.

Mouth-breathing, however, is usually an airway issue. In children, mouth-breathing is often caused by enlarged adenoids or tonsils that are blocking the airway—I refer these patients to an ENT. Sometimes, however, the airway constriction is caused by a mouth that is too small for the tongue. When the palate is not wide enough for the tongue, the tongue rests in the back of the mouth.

**Constricted airway.** Obstructive sleep apnea (OSA) in children can sometimes be successfully treated with expansion therapy at an early age, if the constriction is because the mouth is too small for the tongue. Widening the palate, bringing the teeth forward, and even straightening the teeth, are all ways to make more room for the tongue and prevent it from obstructing the airway.

As I explained in chapter 2, the CBCT 3-D x-ray allows me to see the child's airway and identify any constrictions. It has a color-coded readout that lets me locate the constrictions and the air volume in those areas. That helps me determine whether to pursue an orthodontic solution or to refer the issue out to another specialist.

Often, the parents of a young patient will share with me some symptoms that they're seeing in their child, which also helps me to identify an airway obstruction and potentially obstructive sleep apnea. Some of the symptoms they share include:

- Snoring. Often, a parent will tell me their child breathes very loudly or snores during sleep. If a child snores, they probably have OSA. It's not normal at all for a child to snore, so that's a red flag that OSA is probably present.

- Irritable mornings. When a child is irritable in the morning, there's a good chance it's because they did not get enough sleep the night before, which could be caused by OSA.

- Bedwetting. There are a number of theories as to why OSA causes bedwetting in children, ranging from disruption in the body's signals to the brain that control a child's bladder, to triggering false signals that it's time to "go."

- Behavior issues or poor performance in school. When children don't get enough sleep at night, they tend to misbehave or fall behind in school. It's not that they're purposely behaving badly; it's that they're simply trying to stay awake. And it's not that they're slow learners or poor performers; it's simply that they're too sleepy to keep up.

**Midline discrepancy**. Midline discrepancy is when the upper or lower teeth don't line up in the middle of the face or line up with each other. Typically, at age seven or eight, permanent incisors and four lower permanent incisors are in, but the rest of the teeth are still baby teeth.

Correcting a midline discrepancy is much easier to do before all the permanent teeth have erupted and all the spaces are closed. When there is still space available, the midline can be shifted to the center. Once all the permanent teeth have erupted, it's very difficult to move all the teeth over to one side.

While the aforementioned are problems that can occur, many children don't need early treatment. As mentioned earlier, if a patient is not in need of treatment, I monitor their growth and development every six to twelve months until their permanent teeth have erupted. There is no charge for the first screening visit and the subsequent "growth observation" visits, as they are known, are also free of charge.

## Adolescent Treatment

When children reach adolescence, the goal is for any orthodontics to be their final treatment, whether they had early treatment or not.

Adolescent treatment takes place around ages nine to fourteen, when most of the baby teeth are gone and many permanent teeth have erupted.

One of the main goals in adolescent treatment is to straighten the patient's teeth and give them their best smile. During adolescent treatment, we also correct many jaw growth problems, correct any impacted teeth, and then align the teeth into a good occlusion or bite. Treatment then ends with retainers, which I will discuss in chapter 7. If everything that needs to be corrected is done so as an adolescent, and retainer protocol is followed, then the patient should not need braces or Invisalign as an adult.

A very small percentage of patients that undergo early treatment do not need treatment as an adolescent—but again, that's a small percentage.

## Issues Treated in Adolescence

As with all ages of treatment, there are certain issues that are more treatable in adolescence.

**Spaces or gaps in front teeth**. Normally, when the upper incisors erupt and the other teeth push them together, that movement closes a gap in between the two front teeth. But sometimes, that doesn't happen. Since the problem is so prominent, being in the two front teeth, then most patients want it corrected. That's what they come in reporting as their chief complaint or main concern—the gap in between their front teeth.

**Missing teeth**. Lateral incisors, or the teeth next to the two front teeth, are commonly missing in an adolescent mouth. There are a number of factors that determine how a missing tooth, such as a lateral incisor, is treated. Treatment may involve moving another tooth into the space and then reshaping that tooth. Or, it may include holding the space open and then having an implant placed—implant treatment is only done once all of the facial growth is complete. Moving teeth is sometimes more preferable, because it eliminates the ongoing maintenance and expense of implants. But sometimes, moving a tooth into a space is not the ideal solution, because the shape of the tooth is so different and no amount of reshaping will make it work.

**Impacted teeth**. Again, dealing with impacted teeth may mean moving teeth out of the way so that permanent teeth can come in. That involves using braces or Invisalign to open up the space where the tooth is supposed to erupt, while moving the roots of adjacent teeth out of the way. After a few months of treatment, I take another x-ray, and if it looks like the impacted tooth is moving into the mouth, then we'll wait for it to come in. If the tooth is still impacted regardless of what I do, then the patient is referred to an oral surgeon, who goes under the gum tissue to expose the tooth and place a brace on it. A gold chain is then attached to the brace, and that is used to guide the tooth into the space. Usually, I give the tooth three to six months to erupt once the braces or Invisalign treatment has begun before committing to oral surgery.

**Implants**. Implants are not considered until all the permanent teeth are in and the patient has finished growing. That's because upper teeth continue to grow down until the mouth is fully developed. If an implant is placed at too young an age, the other teeth will continue to grow past the implant, making the implant appear shorter.

If it's determined that an implant is the solution for a space in an adolescent's teeth, then Invisalign or braces are used to create enough space in the teeth, to upright the roots of adjacent teeth, and to correct any other issues.

To hold the space open, the orthodontist places a temporary replacement tooth, known as a pontic, in the space. Once active treatment is complete, a retainer is made with a pontic, so the patient doesn't have to deal with the embarrassment of an unsightly space.

Finally, when all growth has occurred, an oral surgeon places the implant in the patient's jaw, and then the dentist places a crown—the tooth part of the implant—on top of the implant.

An implant is one type of treatment that requires a coordinated effort between multiple providers. For instance, as part of treatment planning the orthodontist, oral surgeon, and general dentist must work together to ensure a success.

**Malocclusions**. Any malocclusions that are correctable in adolescence—such as open bite, deep bite, overbite, underbite, overjet—are treated during these years, because there it is still easier to move teeth and, to some extent, jaws at this age than in adult years. I explained these malocclusions in detail in chapter 3.

**Wisdom teeth**. Not everyone needs their wisdom teeth extracted. To determine whether that is needed, I use the i-CAT FLX CBCT 3-D x-ray to image the jaws to see whether there is enough room for them to erupt in the mouth. If they are already impacted, I recommend that they be removed. If it looks like there might be enough room, then I emphasize the importance of the patient wearing their retainers once treatment is complete. Retainers prevent the wisdom teeth from pushing forward and causing the rest of the newly aligned teeth to become crooked. Stop wearing the retainers, and the erupting wisdom teeth will make the other teeth become crooked faster.

Once all the teeth have come in and the jaw has fully developed, then it can be more difficult to correct problems in the mouth. Still, more adults are seeking treatment today, because either their parents couldn't afford it for them as a teenager, or they've seen changes in their teeth since becoming an adult. Their main concerns are whether treatment will be painful, how it will look on their teeth, how long treatment will last, and, of course, the cost. The next chapter discusses the special issues adults face since movements are more difficult now that growth is complete.

# CHAPTER SIX

# TREATMENT FOR ADULTS

More and more adults are seeking orthodontic treatment. They want to have their best smile, and for many, it has been a lifetime desire.

There are a number of reasons adults seek treatment, but they often come in with several concerns. They want to know if the treatment will be painful, sometimes because they had treatment in the past and remember the pain of those older technologies. They're concerned about how they'll look with braces on their teeth. Many of them want to have straight teeth, but they want to avoid the "look" of metal braces. Some adults have jobs that are in the public eye, so appearance is a concern for them. Then there are athletes and other people with jobs that may occasionally cause them to experience a blow to the face—they want to avoid the injuries that can be caused by braces. Adults also want to know how long the treatment will take, because they have such busy schedules. Costs of treatment, of course, also factor into their decision to have treatment.

Many adults seek orthodontic treatment because they desire a more youthful appearance. As I explained previously, facial features change with age. Most notably, the nose enlarges, the chin grows, and the volume of the face shifts downward as the arches of the mouth tend to shrink in. Teeth also get more crooked with age, and because the teeth support the lips, any changes in the position of the teeth will affect the lips and face.

*Many adults seek orthodontic treatment because they desire a more youthful appearance.*

These issues can be addressed at a very early age by, for instance, ensuring the front teeth remain forward to continue to give the lips support as the person ages. But even in adults, orthodontic treatment can help bring back a youthful smile. By straightening a person's teeth and widening their arches, we can make changes to the skeletal structures of the face that give the lips and cheeks more support and make the face appear rounder. Particularly with lips, if the front teeth are moved forward, the lips move forward, too.

People sometimes have Botox injections for wrinkles around their mouth, but that's a temporary fix. Some have injections to add fullness to their lips. By aligning the teeth and positioning them more forward, the patient's lips gain the long-term support they need to look younger. Orthodontists have the ability to change the structure of the mouth and the positions of the teeth. That can help address wrinkles and make dramatic, permanent improvements in the patient's profile, bringing back some of that youthful appearance. We can make these changes with braces or Invisalign.

However, moving teeth in adults is a more complicated process, compounded by the special issues in the adult mouth. In addition to the changes to the face as a result of aging, adult teeth often need dental procedures to restore their health, before undergoing orthodontic treatment to move everything into place.

Some of the problems that can complicate treatment in adults include:

**Gum disease**. Adults are more likely to have some form of gum disease, which can further complicate or even prevent orthodontic treatment. Gum disease can lead to bone loss in the jaw, weakening the foundation for teeth and placing the health of your smile at risk for the long-term. Additionally, regular dental cleanings combined with a comprehensive oral hygiene routine at home are necessary to ensure optimal oral health during treatment.

**Cracked, chipped, or worn teeth.** As an adult, teeth have had more time to work against each other and cause wear. Often, that means the teeth are cracked or even worn down. I've mentioned bruxism, or clenching and grinding, as one issue many people have. Bruxing can be the result of stress, a health issue such as chronic upset stomach, or just a nervous habit. The problem with bruxing is that, for most people, it occurs only during sleep. So, often, people don't even know they're doing it.

As an adult, if nothing has been done to address that problem and protect the teeth, then there will likely be some level of wear and possibly other damage, such as chipping or fractures, in the teeth. One adult had worn down several of her teeth, to the point of having only the shell of the tooth left above the gumline, by the time she came to me for treatment. Ninety-five percent of several teeth were worn away, and no one had ever made a protective appliance for her to wear.

Teeth can also be chipped, cracked, or worn for other reasons, such as bad habits like nail biting or pencil chewing, accidents such as falls, or from biting into something hard, like ice or popcorn hulls.

**The fully developed jaw** means treatment can no longer take advantage of growth. Healthy teeth can be moved at any age. But in adults, there are no longer opportunities to take advantage of the rapid, natural development of the teeth and jaws. As an adult, the growth of jaws and teeth is complete. That means any misalignments in the jaw structure are more difficult to correct and can take more time.

**Missing teeth**. Missing teeth in adult mouths are more complicated to deal with, in part because teeth don't move as easily in adult bones—so all the movements that have to happen to replace a missing tooth are more complicated. Once a tooth has been missing for some time, then adjacent teeth may tilt into the open space.

Since teeth are always trying to erupt into each other, another problem with missing teeth is that the opposing teeth can grow longer, in an effort to fill the space. For instance, if a back molar has been extracted from the lower jaw, then the opposing molar in the upper jaw may have grown down and appear to be significantly longer than the other upper teeth. Orthodontic treatment must address how to push that upper molar back up or how to otherwise deal with it to align the bite.

## Common Correctable Issues

Issues that are seen in the adult mouth occur largely because there's just been so much more time involved. For example, if someone has had a bad bite, where their teeth aren't coming together correctly, that can lead to a lot of wear and tear and cause teeth to move more over time.

Here are some of the common orthodontic issues we see with adults, and some of the treatments involved in correcting them.

**Crowding, crooked teeth**. This is one of the more common problems we see. Many adults have told me that their teeth were perfectly straight until they were in their thirties or forties, and then their teeth start to shift. Crowding, of course, leads to crooked teeth.

When crowding is corrected as an adult, the newly aligned teeth give the lips more support, making them appear fuller. That's a desirable trait for adults because one of sign of aging, as I mentioned earlier, is where the nose and chin appear larger, but the lips appear thinner. Orthodontic treatment can give the lips more support and create a more youthful appearance.

In many more cases today, because of current advances, crowding can be corrected in an adult without having to extract teeth to make more room. In the past, extractions were the norm to correct crowding and make enough room for the teeth in the mouth. Crowding can be corrected with the newer braces that we use, or with Invisalign.

**Dark triangles** are more prominent in adult teeth. They appear where the teeth meet the gumline, because teeth are typically shaped like triangles and any recession of gum tissue can make the space appear larger. When the teeth are crooked, the tissue can recede and then, when the teeth are straightened, the gap is more apparent because the gum tissue no longer fills the void. There are options I use to minimize the space and make it less noticeable, such as tipping the roots of the teeth toward that space, and sometimes reshaping the teeth.

**Airway issues**. When there is an airway issue in an adult, it is often caused by a mouth that is too small for the tongue.

Using braces or Invisalign, we can make more room for the tongue by aligning the teeth and, to some degree, widening the jaw at the back of the mouth. For extreme cases, orthognathic surgery may help eliminate wearing a CPAP, or continuous positive airway pressure machine. A CPAP is usually prescribed for patients with moderate to severe cases of obstructive sleep apnea. The machine feeds air through a tube and into a mask that the obstructive sleep apnea (OSA) sufferer wears during sleep. While a CPAP is a lifesaving device for patients with OSA, it's also a difficult one for many patients to wear night after night.

Sometimes the mouth is too small for the tongue because of extractions that were done in the past. In extreme cases involving previous extractions, we can use braces or Invisalign to open up the space where the teeth were extracted and then replace those missing teeth with implants. This is a somewhat drastic solution, but not as drastic as jaw surgery. The result is more volume inside the mouth for the tongue, eliminating its tendency to rest in the back of the mouth and obstruct the airway.

**Midline discrepancies**. Adults often want to address a midline discrepancy, but these are far more difficult to correct once the mouth is fully developed. In adults, correcting a midline discrepancy often means performing interproximal reduction (IPR) by removing small amounts of tooth enamel from between the teeth. Even those small amounts can make enough room to move the row of teeth to one side or the other to correct the discrepancy.

## Faster Treatment with Less Pain

As I mentioned, one of the concerns many adults have is how long the treatment will last. At the end of chapter 2, I discussed the micropulse technology and a more invasive procedure that can be performed to accelerate orthodontics. But with the number of advances that are still in the early stages of development or use, the future looks very good to drastically cut treatment time, potentially even in half.

The micropulse technology used for accelerated orthodontics reportedly improves comfort for some patients as well. Patients report less pain as a result of the treatment. The micropulse also helps Invisalign aligners seat around the teeth better and makes them feel more comfortable, so there's less pain with the treatment.

**Finishing Touches**. In a really attractive smile, the teeth—and gums—follow a certain path. After the teeth are straight, if the biting edges or front surfaces are uneven, or if the gum tissue covers one tooth more than others, then the line of the smile is disrupted. That's displeasing to the eye.

As part of treatment, there are optional procedures that may be used to give the smile an extra edge. Two that I use are manicuring and gum contouring.

**Manicuring** is what orthodontists know as enameloplasty. When teeth are crooked, they tend to also wear unevenly on the edges. Once they are straightened, that uneven wear becomes more apparent along the front and biting edges of the teeth. Manicuring involves contouring the teeth back to their ideal shape and restoring their youthful appearance. It's a safe, simple, two- to five-minute procedure that makes a tremendous difference in the final esthetic result.

**Gum contouring** is another procedure that can give the smile that extra edge.

When teeth are aligned, some may be moved down, some moved up. As they move, the gum tissue tends to follow the teeth. That can make the gumline appear uneven at the end of treatment—there may be more gum tissue covering one tooth than the other, adjacent teeth. That unevenness can be distracting to an otherwise perfect smile.

Using the diode laser to reshape the gums can correct many issues with unevenness. Depending on the patient's needs, gum contouring may be done midway in treatment or at the end.

I also use the laser to improve what's known as the "clinical crown." The clinical crown is basically the part of the tooth that is showing outside the gumline. In some patients, the gums just naturally cover more of the teeth than is normal. For instance, when the gum covers one-third or one-half of the crown, the tooth looks a lot smaller. In some cases, the patient may be referred to a periodontist, or a gum specialist. In other cases, I will actually reshape the tissue using the diode laser.

Now that I've covered what is involved in achieving the best smile for patients of all ages, let's look at what it means to keep that smile for a lifetime. After doing all the hard work to get to your best smile, it's time to take measures to maintain it.

# CHAPTER SEVEN

# RETAINING YOUR SMILE

For years, orthodontists have tried to develop ways to keep the teeth aligned (straight) following treatment with braces or Invisalign clear aligner therapy. The goal has been to have patients wear their retainers full time for a few months, and thereafter the teeth would stay straight for a lifetime. Unfortunately, it doesn't work that way— teeth refuse to remain stable without wearing retainers for life.

That's because the body is always changing. Jawbones are living structures; they're not static. Teeth have forces on them that cause them to move: that includes pressure from the cheeks, which are always pushing in; pressure from the tongue, which is always pushing out; and clenching and grinding, which is always wearing away at the teeth. So, even patients that had naturally straight teeth when they were younger can end up with crowded or crooked teeth when they get older.

Studies have shown that 90 percent of all patients that have had orthodontic treatment experience a significant relapse of their teeth if they don't wear their retainers.[8] In other words, their teeth tend to move back into the misaligned position they were in before being straightened. Only 10 percent of people treated won't experience any significant relapse without wearing retainers. But since there is currently no way to tell which patients will relapse and which won't, then I treat everyone as someone who needs to wear retainers for life.

*Even patients that had naturally straight teeth when they were younger can end up with crowded or crooked teeth when they get older.*

## Getting Your Retainers

Retainers are ready within a few days or a couple of weeks after braces are removed; it all depends on the tendency for a patient's teeth to move as soon as treatment is finished.

When a patient finishes treatment with braces or Invisalign, we take an intraoral scan of their teeth in order to make new models, now that their teeth are straightened. We then use those digital models to make the retainers.

In the past, we would take an impression of the patient's teeth and send that to the lab. Today, we send in the digital scan, which the lab uses to make the patient's retainers. Those retainers are delivered up to two weeks later.

However, we also have 3-D printers, which allow us to make retainers in-house. That lets us have the retainers available the same or next day for patients that have a greater chance of significant relapse

---

8    Little, RM, Riedel RA, Artun J, "An evaluation of changes in mandibular anterior alignment for 10 to 20 years postretention," American Journal of Orthodontics and Dentofacial Orthopedics, 1988:93: p 423-428.

as soon as their braces are removed. Currently, there is a concern for immediate relapse with maybe 5 percent of my cases, and they are typically patients that had large spaces that were closed, a lot of teeth that were moved, or a significant number of cracked teeth (indicating a lot of clenching). To determine whether there is a greater chance of relapse, I look at the patient's "before" photos and case notes.

But for most patients, any movement once the braces are removed is very gradual, so waiting two weeks for retainers from the lab is not an issue.

One of the plusses of Invisalign is that we can create the digital models at the end of treatment and send them off to the lab, but the patient can continue to wear their aligners until their retainers are ready. With braces, once the wires and brackets are removed, the teeth are free to move until the retainers are available to hold them in place. But I know from experience which teeth are most likely to relapse in a hurry; those are the patients I want to put in retainers as quickly as possible. Depending on how urgent the need, we can have the patient in retainers faster now, thanks to the 3-D printer technology.

In the past, every patient of mine was prescribed retainers full-time for about six months. Then, they only had to the wear their retainers at night. But wearing retainers all day made it difficult to speak, and they were often lost when removed for eating and cleaning. So, I tried changing the retention protocol to nighttime-only wear— every night. It didn't take long to realize that nighttime-only was enough time for straightened teeth to remain in place. Since the new protocol was easier on patients' lifestyles, I also found them to be far more cooperative in wearing their retainers. As a result, we've had far better results in patient outcomes over the long term.

## Types of Retainers

There are different types of retainers, and the type used depends on the patient's needs. When a patient's treatment is finished—whether that be with braces or Invisalign—I decide what type of retainer they need for each arch. Sometimes, I prescribe one type of retainer for the upper arch and a different type for the lower arch. Sometimes, they wear the same type on each arch; it all depends on the patient's needs.

**Clear retainers**. The type of retainers I use most often are clear retainers. These are very similar to standard Invisalign aligners, but they are thicker, stronger, and last longer. Clear retainers slide over all the teeth, upper and lower, and are practically invisible. These are removable retainers, intended to be worn only at night.

Since they cover all the teeth, an added advantage of clear retainers is that they also cushion the teeth, protecting them from damage caused by nighttime grinding. That can also help prevent jaw pain. However, this type of retainer is different than a night guard for clenching and grinding, which I will talk about later in this chapter.

**Hawley retainers**. These are acrylic, tongue-shaped retainers that are crafted to fit comfortably in the mouth and be held in place by metal wires that clamp onto the teeth. A fun feature of Hawley retainers is that the acrylic part can be personalized with different colors and patterns—options even include electric or sparkly colors, camouflage or rainbows, or favorite sports teams. An advantage to these retainers is that, if the teeth move slightly, I can correct their alignment with the retainer. These are also removable retainers, intended to be worn only at night.

**Fixed retainers**. One type of retainer is actually designed to remain in the mouth at all times. Known as a fixed retainer, this type of retainer is a wire that is bonded to the backside of the front teeth, either on the top or bottom arch, or both.

I rarely use the fixed retainer these days, except with patients that have a space in their front teeth that is prone to opening up during the day when their nighttime retainers are not in. The reasons? The wire tends to break loose at some point, and the wearers rarely realize their wire is no longer attached until their teeth have moved. At that point, it's difficult to realign the teeth without undergoing treatment again. Plus, fixed aligners are hard to floss around and keep clean, which can cause decay and gum disease on the very teeth that were just straightened. Finally, they only keep the front teeth straight; they don't work on the back teeth.

In truth, I'm not a fan of fixed retainers for the reasons I've stated. And usually, after a year of wearing them, patients switch over to removable versions—they simply don't work for most people.

## Caring for Retainers

One reason patients sometimes stop wearing their retainers is because they can get a little, well, grungy. That's because proteins in saliva tend to accumulate on them while they are worn.

The best way to care for retainers is to brush them with a toothbrush and toothpaste after removing them in the morning. Even then, however, they tend to discolor or develop a buildup of calcium. Using a denture cleanser like Efferdent or Polydent once a week can help keep the retainers clean. The cleanser should be used only for a few minutes, per the instructions on the box, as soaking the retainers overnight can make them deteriorate.

Also, keep your retainer in the provided case when it's not in use. Do not leave it on the nightstand (dogs love to chew on the plastic), or take it out at the breakfast table (it can get tossed away in a napkin), as it can get costly to continually replace destroyed or lost retainers.

## Retainer Policy

At my practice, the first set of retainers is included with the orthodontic treatment plan, and that set is guaranteed for one year. After that, there is a charge to replace cracked or broken retainers. There is also a charge for retainers lost in the first year.

With removable retainers, we see patients periodically for the first year after treatment to ensure they are wearing their retainers as instructed and that the retainers are keeping their teeth stable. After the first year, we ask patients to call us if they have issues that need to be addressed. With fixed retainers, we must continually monitor the patient for a lifetime to ensure the retainers stay in place and that the patient isn't developing an oral health problem because of the wire.

Most retainers last for years; I've had patients wear the same retainers for decades. Retainers are a little like glasses: some people wear the same prescription for a long time, some people are constantly breaking their glasses and need a new pair practically every year.

The mouth is a very hostile environment, but retainers are built to take a lot of wear and tear. Still, they can be damaged by serious problems with clenching and grinding. In some cases, a patient may even bite through a clear retainer. At that point, they may need a night guard or splint.

## Night Guards and Splints

When a regular retainer is not enough to keep a patient's teeth straight and protected from the damaging effects of clenching and grinding, I can fashion what's known as a night guard, or splint, that also acts as a retainer. Night guards are made of extra-durable material, which is thicker than a normal retainer, so they can withstand the forces from constant clenching and grinding.

Night guards can also protect the jaws from the detrimental effects of TMJ. That's something I evaluate for when determining what type of retainer a patient needs. Even if a patient doesn't report the typical symptoms of TMJ—jaw pain, clicking and popping noises in the jaw, headaches on waking, "frozen" jaws or jaws stuck in an open or closed position—I may identify the problem by the amount of wear on their teeth. If I see significant wear on their back teeth, I know they're likely dealing with bruxism, or clenching and grinding, during sleep.

There are different types of night guards available depending on the issues the patient has. Night guards are created off-site, in a lab, because they require very specific construction.

## A Lasting Smile

Again, retention is the key to keeping your smile for a lifetime. That applies whether or not you still have wisdom teeth. At the end of treatment, patients often ask me whether their wisdom teeth will cause their teeth to become crooked.

As I mentioned at the end of chapter 5, as part of the evaluation in advance of treatment, I use an

*Retention is the key to keeping your smile for a lifetime.*

x-ray to image the patient's mouth and determine whether there is enough room for all the corrections without having to extract the wisdom teeth. If I don't see any issues, I can correct the teeth and jaws without extracting the wisdom teeth. However, if retainers are not worn nightly as prescribed, the wisdom teeth certainly can contribute to movement in the other teeth, causing them to crowd. In the cases where an x-ray does indicate possible impactions of wisdom teeth, then I refer them to an oral surgeon for evaluation.

Someday, we may very well figure out a way to keep teeth straight without retention. But until that day, the only way to keep your beautiful new smile is by wearing retainers for life.

# CHAPTER EIGHT

# A BETTER EXPERIENCE

Orthodontic treatment today is geared toward a better patient experience overall.

For starters, the technologies today are generally making treatment faster, more comfortable and convenient, less intrusive into a lifestyle, and just a better experience overall.

But as I've mentioned, what really matters is who performs the treatment. There's a lot to be said for the experience guiding the tools during an orthodontic treatment plan. And with that experience comes insight and intuition into what patients need and want with their treatment.

That said, there are a number of factors that set Lindsey Orthodontics apart as a practice that patients choose for their orthodon-

> *There's a lot to be said for the experience guiding the tools during an orthodontic treatment plan.*

tic needs. In this chapter, I'll share with you just a few reasons we have so many referrals.

## A More Comfortable Experience

From the moment you step into Lindsey Orthodontics, you'll notice a difference. Little extras such as music-themed décor, a jukebox playing a few tunes, video games for all ages, free Wi-Fi, and fresh-baked cookies daily, make the office environment relaxing and fun.

Every visit begins with a warm greeting from our truly patient-focused staff. My team has the training and experience to ensure that all your questions are answered and that you understand what you need and want to know about your treatment.

In the first visit, the initial consultation, a patient coordinator will gather background information about the patient and then provide a tour of the office. We also take diagnostic x-rays and photos and conduct a clinical exam in the first consultation, to get a better understanding of the patient's needs. In some patients, we may even take a 3-D scan using the CBCT imaging machine.

Once the tests are completed, I then visit with each patient. I ask the patient (and their parent) about what they envision as their best smile. Then, I evaluate the x-rays and other tests to see what's going on with the patient's teeth, gums, and jaws. Those tests help me determine what we can offer in the way of treatment. I also ask about any symptoms that may indicate the presence of TMJ or an obstruction of the airway; that's need-to-know information to help determine part of the treatment plan.

As I've discussed in previous chapters, depending on the patient's needs, treatment may be recommended right away, or it may be delayed until more development has occurred. If treatment is recommended, I discuss with the patient (and parent) in that first consultation the advantages and disadvantages of treatment options.

If treatment is recommended, our financial coordinator will discuss the various options for payment. These are explained later in this chapter.

## Better Technology

Over time, I have had the pleasure of experiencing how much things have improved in orthodontics since I first started treating patients. As I mentioned earlier, technology has completely changed what we're able to accomplish today, while making the entire treatment experience much better for patients.

Braces and Invisalign are both more efficient at moving teeth, so patients don't have to come in for adjustments as often as in the past. When I first started treating patients, they had to come back for adjustments every four weeks. Now, because of the improvement in the wires we use for braces, they usually only have to come in once every eight weeks. The wires with braces also make the treatment more comfortable, moving teeth with a lighter, more continuous force. That allows treatment to finish in the same or less time than treatments of the past.

With Invisalign, the visits are normally twelve weeks apart. As I mentioned in chapter 4, that's more convenient because it requires less time off from work, school, or other activities. Athletes, cheerleaders, band members, and people in jobs that require a lot of travel, all appreciate that there are fewer visits, farther apart.

As I mentioned, we have intraoral scanners now, which means we don't have to take impressions of teeth with modeling goop anymore. That was the part of orthodontics that many people dreaded the most. Today, we use the scanners to create digital models of the teeth for retainers and for treatment with Invisalign or any of the appliances we use.

As I've mentioned, my offices have 3-D printers, allowing us to create retainers in-office. That's especially important for patients whose teeth are prone to moving once treatment is complete.

We also have the CBCT 3-D x-ray machine, which allows me to see not only the teeth and gums, but also all the underlying structures of the head and neck, including the airway. Those images provide me with the information I need to guide teeth into place, and they also let me know whether the patient has an airway that is so narrow it is causing them problems—whether they know it or not.

## Better Quality

In my practice, quality takes priority over patient numbers. But as a result, we're busy all the time. That's because of patient referrals; the vast majority of my patients come from referrals by other patients. By delivering quality, we are the provider of choice by patients who refer us to their family and friends. So, while I've always been wired to deliver quality treatment, I'm also driven by the fact that it's the reason I'm in business today. Making treatment a pleasant experience for every patient is more than a motivator, it's also very rewarding. I love being able to give patients their best smile, but I'm also rewarded when they tell their family and friends about their experience.

## A Love of Learning

One of the things that sets Lindsey Orthodontics apart is a lifelong love of learning. My formal orthodontic education started at the University of Kentucky. The chairman of the department was Dr. Orhan Tuncay, who instilled in me the importance of critical thinking while studying all areas of orthodontics. I will always be grateful for his acceptance and mentorship. Over the years, my own continuing education has included following the teachings of the strongest influencers in orthodontics. These include Dr. Dwight Damon, developer of an innovative, self-ligating bracket system, and Dr. David Sarver, who has written about macro-, micro-, and mini-esthetics, which are crucial when analyzing facial and dental components in orthodontic treatment planning. I've spent considerable time reading books, attending lectures, and taking courses by these two thought leaders and others, so that I can keep my practices at the forefront of changes in the industry. I have also followed influencers for Invisalign, seeing it as the future of orthodontics. One of my most instrumental instructors in the use and mastery of Invisalign as a treatment tool for orthodontics has been Dr. Willy Dayan of Toronto, Canada. His vast experience and ability to teach the complicated force systems needed to create the patient's best smile in the use of customized clear aligners (Invisalign) is unsurpassed.

What I've learned through all these experiences allows me to offer treatment that is light years ahead of where the industry was during my residency as an orthodontist some thirty years ago.

We also believe in ongoing learning at my practice, where team members participate in education through in-house training on clinical-, patient-, and business-oriented topics designed to continually improve the overall orthodontic experience.

## The Brace Bus

One of the challenges of orthodontic treatment has been fitting the periodic appointments into a busy lifestyle. That's especially important for parents, who often must take off work to bring their child in. It's also an issue for kids, however, who must take off time from school or miss practice for their extracurricular activities. Again, the technologies now require fewer appointments. But another feature we offer makes it even easier to get to and from appointments.

The Brace Bus is an H-2 Hummer that we use to transport students from area schools to their appointment. Once their appointment is finished, we transport them back to school. The service is complimentary and allows students to be excused for their appointment without losing credit for the school day.

## Financing for Treatment

How to finance treatment is one of the concerns that most adults have, whether for their child or themselves. We have options today that make financing easier for patients. Our goal is to make treatment accessible to everyone. We never want finances to be a hurdle to having your best smile.

*Our goal is to make treatment accessible to everyone.*

As I mentioned at the end of chapter 1, the cost of orthodontics is very affordable today. In fact, comparatively speaking, the cost of having orthodontic treatment has not really increased over time.

To help make treatment affordable, we offer a number of payment plans and options. We take cash, checks, and credit cards for payment, and offer discounts for paying in full upfront. When patients have dental insurance that covers orthodontic treatment, we gladly go over their policy to help determine coverage, file the claims, and accept assignment. At Lindsey Orthodontics, we offer our in-house financing with no interest charged.

We also have low- and no-interest financing available through a third-party credit system. These plans typically require no down payment, and payment schedules can extend even beyond the completion of treatment.

Each month, we also have specials available that offer discounts for starting treatment. These can sometimes make it more affordable to start treatment now, rather than waiting.

There is one other factor that sets Lindsey Orthodontics apart and that goes beyond providing quality orthodontic care and improving smiles. We believe in improving our community. In the next chapter, I'll discuss ways in which we give back in thanks for all the good that's come our way.

# CHAPTER NINE

# GIVING BACK

I have been very fortunate to have had a great career in orthodontics. As a result, I feel compelled to give back as a sort of repayment for all the good that has come my way. When I give back, the activities I focus on center around my profession, dentistry and orthodontics, and my personal passion, aviation.

*I feel compelled to give back as a sort of repayment for all the good that has come my way.*

I mentioned in the introduction how my love of aviation started at a young age. My father was a maintenance foreman at Eastern Airlines, so I've always been around airplanes. My first aspiration for a career was to be a commercial airline pilot, but at age seven I found out I was nearsighted. Since LASIK surgery wasn't available then, being a commercial pilot wasn't going to be an option. Still, when I was twenty, I had a chance to fly with a pilot in a two-seater airplane and that sealed the deal. I earned my private pilot's license at Georgia Tech through its flying club. That was in 1977, and I've been flying ever since.

I had only thirteen hours of flying when I first soloed a plane. That was a real eye-opening experience, to look over and see an empty seat where an instructor had always been. Now, I've been flying for more than four decades, and as you can probably tell, I still enjoy every flight. Over the years, there have been a number of very exciting trips. It was beautiful to fly over the Bahamas on the way down to Turks and Caicos. And as I was writing this book, I went to Florida and flew seaplanes with a friend. It was amazing to take off and land from the water, and to fly only a couple of hundred feet above the water, enjoying the sights of beautiful houses, boats, and alligators.

My own airplane is a Beechcraft Baron, a twin-engine piston aircraft with 260-horsepower engine on each wing. It flies around two hundred miles per hour, with four people and all of their luggage. I use it, of course, to fly my family on vacation, but I also use it for a number of other purposes.

## Sharing the Love of Flying with Others

I feel very fortunate to live in a country with all of the freedoms we enjoy. I exercise that right through my love of flying. Whether I'm flying my family somewhere on vacation, giving patients a ride, or taking a young aviator on their first flight, I share my love for aviation by encouraging others to get involved in the industry.

There is a developing shortage for pilots in the corporate and commercial areas of the airline industry. Many longtime pilots are retiring, and it's becoming difficult to get young pilots interested in flying—in part because the training is so costly. But we need good, qualified pilots in the air if we're going to ensure the future of the industry.

That's why I enjoy participating in the Young Eagles of the Experimental Aircraft Association (EAA). I am the Young Eagles coordinator for the local chapter and we have three events each year, through which pilots encourage interest in flight for our youth. Many of the youth we take up on private planes have never flown on any type of airplane. But by sharing our interest in aviation, we hope that some will ultimately pursue aviation careers. In fact, several of those that I have given rides to as part of the program have gone into aviation as a career. That's a very rewarding feeling for me.

The Young Eagles events are for youth ages eight to seventeen. The events involve an orientation to general aviation and a ride-along with a pilot. Then the youth are given a certificate and a logbook as evidence of their flight. Usually, more than fifty kids attend the event and experience that first exciting flight.

The events can be very motivating for young people, whether they want to be a pilot, a mechanic, or work in management or some other area of aviation. I remember one young lady in particular. Kayla flew with me when she was fourteen, and I later found out that flight inspired her to join a Youth Program in which participants learn to work on airplanes. Today, she has her private pilot's license and is planning a career in aviation. And she attributes it all to her first flight in Young Eagles. So the program does work. It benefits the young people that get involved, but it also benefits aviation to have quality people take an interest in the industry.

The local events are part of a national program that has flown more than one million children to date.

As I mentioned in the last chapter, I have a love of learning in orthodontics and dentistry. That applies to aviation as well. Since

I earned my license, I have continued to earn more flight ratings. Today, I have a commercial rating, an instrument rating, which allows me to fly through clouds, a seaplane rating, and an instructor's rating for single- and multi-engine airplanes. Many of these ratings I've sought just because I wanted to be a better pilot. The instructor rating, in particular, was really just to get me to that level of airmanship where I would be the best possible pilot for my family and for the people I fly.

## Angel Flights

Another way I give back as a pilot is by helping to transport patients over large distances through the Angel Flight organization. This is an organization that connects private pilots with patients who need to travel long distances for a test, treatment, a hospital stay, or other medical need. The patients are transported free of charge; the plane and fuel are donated by the pilots.

Sometimes, patients are traveling such a long distance that it takes several flights in single-engine aircraft to fly them to and from their destination. Since I have a faster airplane, I'm often able to transport patients from farther away in a single flight. That was the case with one chemotherapy patient who needed treatment from a provider in a neighboring state. She and her husband met me at the airport, where he explained that he could no longer afford to take off work, because they needed his income to pay for, among other things, her mounting medical bills.

Other patients that I fly need surgery or are visiting a specialist for treatment for a very rare medical condition. For instance, a specialist in Atlanta has developed a helmet to help reshape a child's misshapen head. But that helmet has to be adjusted about every two weeks. That's a considerable drive and inconvenience, as well as a financial hardship, for people that live in neighboring states. Being able to take a one-hour flight is so much more convenient than the time off work and the expense of a six- or seven-hour drive in their car.

I've been flying patients through Angel Flight for twenty years now. It has been as rewarding of an experience for me as it is for the people I fly. They never fail to express their deep appreciation for the help at a difficult time in their lives.

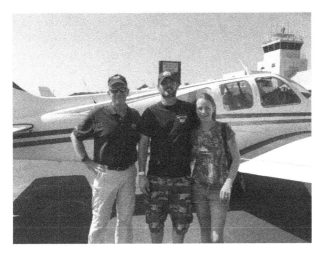

*Dr. Lindsey volunteers for a charitable organization called Angel Flight. He's flown patients in need of medical attention to various medical treatment centers in the United States.*

## Patient Appreciation Day

Every year, my practice holds a Patient Appreciation Day at a local airport. The event has often been catered by a local restaurant, The Varsity, which serves up hamburgers, hot dogs, French fries, and other treats. We also bring in a vendor that serves slushy drinks and ice cream.

All kinds of fun takes place at the event: music, face painting, and photographs taken in costumes, are just a few of the activities that we've had.

The highlight of the event is when I take patients and their families for a ride in my airplane. When the weather is good, it's not unusual to me to take more than 100 patients on a ride during the event. For some patients, it's the first time they've flown and it creates a memory they will have forever.

## Giving Back Through Dentistry

I also like to give back through my profession, and one way I do that is through the Hope Health Clinic in Griffin, Georgia. Hope Health Clinic provides medical and dental care for patients at no charge.

Among the patients at Hope Health are young children that need orthodontic treatment, but whose families can't afford to pay for it. These are young children that care about their teeth, and they show it by brushing and taking good care of them. The dentists that work at Hope Health Clinic screen these patients for me and select which ones they think would benefit from orthodontic treatment. They look for children that would really benefit from having their best smile throughout their life.

As a way of giving back, I provide orthodontic treatment at no cost for these select patients. Those that I've treated have been very appreciative—their parents often show up at my practice with baked goods or other small gifts. As an example of the success of this program, one young man from a disadvantaged family has graduated from high school, and is now attending school at a major university.

He attributes his successes to the confidence he's gained from having straight teeth and his best smile.

Providing such patients with their best smile is far more rewarding to me than just making financial donations. I would rather give back by using my skills to try to better patients' lives, and fortunately, programs like the one through Hope Health Clinic help me in doing so.

My practice also awards scholarships every year to patients that graduate from high school, as a way of helping them continue their education. The scholarships are granted to teens that write an essay explaining their financial situation, why they want to go on to college, and what they hope to accomplish with their studies. We have dozens of applications each year, and the number keeps increasing. To date, we've given out over $30,000 in scholarships.

In addition to the aforementioned activities, Lindsey Orthodontics is always looking for ways to give back to show patients—and our communities—how much we appreciate them. We want everyone to know how thankful we are that they chose us to help them achieve their best smile.

# CONCLUSION

Having read my book, I hope you now have a good idea of how exciting the field of orthodontics has become and what it can do for the lives of people that pursue treatment. I hope you become as excited about the options available to you today as I am in being able to offer them to you.

I've been extremely fortunate to have chosen an enjoyable career in an industry that has seen tremendous—and positive—changes since I began treating patients more than three decades ago. It is extremely rewarding to see the dramatic results that modern orthodontics makes possible. As an orthodontist, I love being able to help patients obtain their best smiles, and I love seeing those smiles improve their self-confidence and their lives.

My team and I have seen that happen time and again. A patient comes in for an initial consult. At first, quite often, they're reserved and sometimes a little shy. Sometimes, they don't even want to show us their teeth. That happens with children and adults. But before the visit is over, they already seem to feel more comfortable with their surroundings and are more assured by the welcome they have received. Treatment is recommended, but sometimes there are concerns about financing. We talk through the various options and find that treatment can fit into the budget. Already, they begin to feel better just because something is being done about their smile. Another visit or two, and they begin to really open up—they share stories with us about their treatment, their family and friends, their school or job, their lives. By the time treatment is complete, they are a different person—happy and outgoing and smiling for all the world to see.

Remember, your smile is your best asset. It can make you more confident, and that can help you make friends, get a job, find a mate, and be remembered. With a great smile, you are also likely to have better health. In short, that one simple gesture—smiling—can make all the difference.

If you've been dreaming about the difference a beautiful smile can make, now is the time to turn your dreams into reality. With the advances in treatment today, we can help you have a happier, healthier smile—*your* best smile—for life.

# APPENDIX

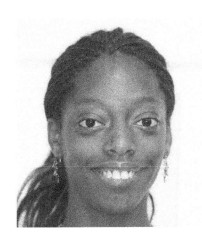 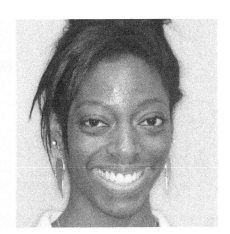

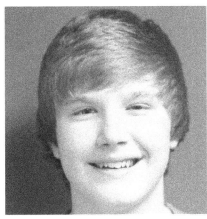 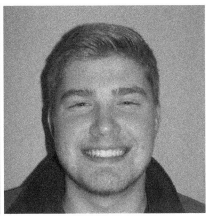

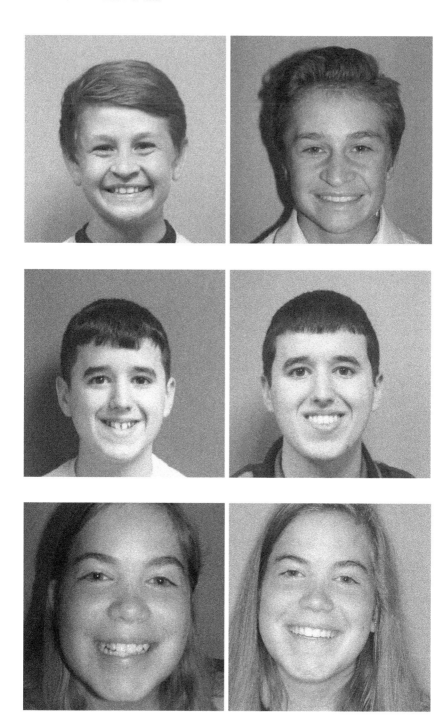

# GLOSSARY

**3-D printer**. These are used to print out the models of the teeth from the image sent from the 3-D scanner. The models can be used to make various appliances and retainers.

**3-D scanner**. The 3-D scanner eliminates the need for a tray of "goop" to make an impression of the teeth, which was used a mold of the mouth. 3-D scanners allow for digital models of the mouth to the be made.

**abnormal eruptions**. Abnormal eruptions, also known as ectopic eruptions, are teeth that erupt out of position in the mouth. An abnormal eruption can occur almost anywhere in the mouth.

**alastics**. Elastic bands or rings that fit around the braces. In some offices they are used to hold the archwire into the bracket. Our brackets have "doors" that hold the archwire in place. We use alastics as a decoration on the braces if the patient desires them.

**anterior**. The front of the mouth.

**arch**. The shape of the row of teeth in the upper or lower jaw.

**attachments**. Clear-colored bumps that are bonded directly to the teeth as part of treatment with Invisalign clear aligners. Each attachment is specifically designed to provide the necessary grip to help the aligners push on the teeth to move them in the desired direction.

**bruxism**. Clenching and grinding of the teeth.

**canines**. The teeth next to the incisors (the four front teeth).

**clinical crown**. This is the part of the tooth that shows outside the gumline; it is the part of the tooth that people see.

**cone beam computed tomography (CBCT)**. A type of very low-dose x-ray machine that produces 3-D images of the soft and hard tissues of the face and neck.

**constricted airway**. This is a narrowing of the airway due to an obstruction, which can lead to obstructive sleep apnea (OSA).

**crossbite**. A malocclusion where the upper teeth are inside the lower teeth during a bite, leading to abnormal tooth wear, biting trauma to the teeth, or serious gum problems.

**crowding or crooked teeth**. This condition occurs when there is not enough room for the teeth to erupt during development. Crowding is unattractive and can increase the risk for tooth decay and gum disease because it's harder to keep teeth clean.

**diode laser**. The diode laser is used to expose teeth that are having trouble erupting and to contour gum tissue to make the gums look more symmetric.

**elastics (rubber bands)**. These are attached to the lower and upper braces to correct how the teeth fit together. They must be changed out by the patient throughout treatment.

**embrasure**. The small, v-shaped space between teeth at the biting edges.

**ENT**. Ear, nose, and throat specialist.

**expander**. An appliance that is used to widen the upper palate in young patients.

**general dentist**. These professionals offer a wide range of services including regular checkups, cleanings, dental fillings, crowns, bridges, crowns on implants, teeth whitening, extractions, and more. They work with orthodontists and other specialists to provide comprehensive dental care.

**gum contouring**. A procedure using a diode laser to make the gums more symmetric.

**gummy smile**. A condition in which too much of the gum tissue shows during a smile.

**habit appliances**. These are used to correct bad oral habits such as thumb-sucking and tongue thrust, which can lead to development issues that could require extensive treatment to correct.

**Herbst appliance**. A stainless-steel bar that is fixed to the braces on the upper and lower teeth on the side of the mouth and helps guide growth of the jaw.

**impacted tooth**. This is a tooth that is not erupting into the mouth as expected.

**incisors**. The four teeth in the front/center of the smile.

**Interproximal Reduction (IPR)**. A process that involves mechanically removing very small amounts of tooth enamel in between the teeth to create room for straightening them.

**Invisalign**. Clear aligners that are used to move teeth. Often chosen as a treatment option over traditional braces.

**lateral incisors**. The teeth next to the two front teeth.

**malocclusion**. A bad bite.

**manicuring**. Known by orthodontists as enameloplasty, manicuring is a safe, simple procedure that involves contouring the teeth back to their ideal shape and restoring their youthful appearance.

**maxillary**. Referring to the upper jaw.

**micropulse technology**. A type of technology that uses vibration to stimulate the teeth and help them move faster.

**mismatched dental midlines**. A mismatched midline is when the upper and lower front teeth don't meet in the middle. This is easier to correct in children, before all the teeth have erupted.

**mouth-breathing**. In children, this may be caused by enlarged adenoids or tonsils that are blocking the airway. It may also be caused by a mouth that is too small for the tongue, causing the tongue to rest in the back of the mouth and block the airway.

**occlusion**. The bite. There are three classes of bites: class I (a good bite), class II (a bite where the upper teeth are more forward than the lower teeth), and class III (a bite where the lower teeth are more forward than the upper teeth).

**obstructive sleep apnea (OSA).** A condition where the person actually periodically stops breathing while sleeping. This can cause a multitude of serious physical problems and even death.

**open bite.** In an open bite, the front teeth don't meet. Open bite can be the result of development, tongue thrust, or bad habits like thumb-sucking.

**oral surgeon.** This is a specialist that deals with problems that require surgical treatment such as orthognathic (jaw) surgery, exposing impacted teeth, placing implants, and extracting wisdom teeth.

**orthognathic surgery.** Jaw surgery.

**overbite (or deep bite).** The upper front teeth overlap the lower front teeth, concealing the lower front teeth when the smile is viewed from the front.

**overjet (or upper front teeth protrusion).** This bite is characterized by the upper teeth extending too far forward or the lower teeth not extending far enough forward.

**OSA.** See obstructive sleep apnea.

**pediatric dentist.** This is a dental specialist for children.

**periodontist.** This is a specialist that treats problems with gum tissue and the bone that surrounds the teeth.

**posterior.** The back of the mouth.

**quad helix.** An expander appliance that applies gentle force to the upper palate to reshape the jaw over about a six- to eight-month period.

**refinements**. This takes place during treatment with Invisalign clear aligners and involves taking another scan, ordering another set of aligners, removing the attachments as needed and placing new ones to finish up the case.

**self-ligating.** Self-ligating braces have a door that holds the wire in place. With self-ligating braces, there is less friction and binding of the wire in the brackets.

**SmartTrack**. The unique, patented, dual-layer plastic that Invisalign clear aligners are made of.

**space maintainers.** These help to hold space open when baby teeth have fallen out or when a child has lost their baby teeth very early.

**spacing**. Sometimes known as gaps. Although not typically a health problem, gaps in teeth can ruin an otherwise beautiful smile.

**TMD or TMJ**. Temporomandibular joint disfunction. Refers to a broad range of problems associated with the jaw joint.

**tongue thrust**. The tongue chronically pushing through the front teeth, potentially creating an open bite.

**underbite**. When the lower teeth jut out farther than the upper teeth, which can cause abnormal teeth wear, poor chewing, and an unsightly smile.

# OUR SERVICES

At Lindsey Orthodontics, we want patients to know that we care about their needs, and we work hard to answer all of their questions and concerns. Our ongoing training and experience, combined with the latest technologies and techniques in orthodontics, ensure patients receive a smile that is both beautiful and functional. After all, that's why we're here—to make a positive difference by giving every patient their best smile.

Services we offer include:

- Early treatment for children

- Adolescent treatment

- Adult treatment

- Palatal expansion

- Thumb-habit appliances

- Damon metal and clear braces

- Invisalign

- Retainers

- Digital technologies

- Brace Bus

Reach out to us at:

## Griffin Office

120 W. College St., Suite A

Griffin, Georgia 30224

Phone: 770-228-1223

## Locust Grove Office

4600 Bill Gardner Parkway, Suite 100

Locust Grove, Georgia 30248

Phone: 770-914-7994

www.lindseyorthodontics.com

CPSIA information can be obtained
at www.ICGtesting.com
Printed in the USA
LVHW080744101019
633650LV00032B/1821/P